TAROT
FOR
PREGNANCY

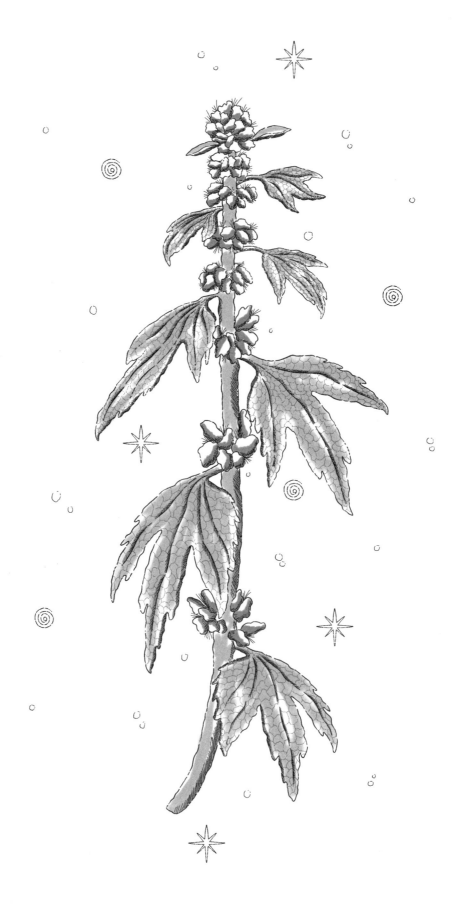

TAROT
FOR
PREGNANCY

A Companion for
Radical Magical Birthing Folks

BRITTANY CARMONA-HOLT
THE BIRTH WITCH

Library of Congress Cataloging-in-Publication Data Available Upon Request

ISBN 978-1-955905-03-9 (TP)

Ebook ISBN: 978-1-955905-17-6

Printed in the United States

Cover and interior illustrations by Kimberly Rodriguez

Cover lettering by Kaylee Agnello

Book Design by Pauline Neuwirth, Neuwirth & Associates, Inc.

Distributed by Simon & Schuster

First edition

10 9 8 7 6 5 4 3 2 1

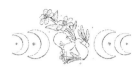

CONTENTS

Welcome   xi

How to Use This Book   xv

Glossary of Terms   xvii

THE HISTORY [MYSTERY] OF THE TAROT   5
by Sanyu Estelle Nagenda, "The Word Witch"

A NOTE ON REVERSALS   17

A NOTE ON REPEATING CARDS   21

THE MINOR ARCANA:
CONCEPTION-BIRTH

**THE ACES—MONTH 1: MENSTRUAL CYCLE TO THE
FIRST TWO WEEKS OF PREGNANCY (WEEKS 1 TO 4)**   27

    JOURNAL: Begin Tracking Your Emotional Journey   32

    RECIPE: Nausea Tea   39

THE TWOS—MONTH 2 (WEEKS 5 TO 8)   42

    JOURNAL: Self-Reflection through Relationship   44

    TAROT SPREAD: Choosing a Health Care Provider   46

THE THREES—MONTH 3 (WEEKS 9 TO 13)   49

    EXERCISE: Brainstorming for Village Building   51

    RECIPE: Nourishing Pregnancy Infusion   55

THE FOURS—MONTH 4 (WEEKS 14 TO 17)   58

    JOURNAL: The Pause   62

    TAROT SPREAD: Honing Intuition and Removing Self-Limiting Blockages   66

THE FIVES—MONTH 5 (WEEKS 18 TO 21)   67

  RECIPE: Herbal Tea for Heartburn and Digestion   72

THE SIXES—MONTH 6 (WEEKS 22 TO 26)   73

  EXERCISE: Detoxifying Cleanse   75

  JOURNAL: Detoxifying   76

THE SEVENS—MONTH 7 (WEEKS 27 TO 30)   80

  JOURNAL: Document Your Emotional Experience   82

  EXERCISE: Clearing Your Intuition from Doubtful Voices   84

  RECIPE: Soothing Belly Rub   86

THE EIGHTS—MONTH 8 (WEEKS 31 TO 35)   89

  JOURNAL: Release   92

  EXERCISE: Visualize Speaking Your Truth   94

  TAROT SPREAD: Letting Go   95

THE NINES—MONTH 9 (WEEKS 36 TO 40)   96

  JOURNAL: Nearing the End of Pregnancy   98

  SUGGESTED PACKING LIST FOR AN OUT-OF-HOME BIRTH BAG   103

THE TENS—FINAL WEEKS OF PREGNANCY, BIRTH, AND POSTPARTUM   105

  JOURNAL: Processing and Integrating Your Birth Story   109

  A LITTLE NOTE FOR BIRTH PARTNERS AND DOULAS   113

  RECIPE: Herbal Sitz Bath Tea   116

  RECIPE: Nutritious Herbal Infusion for Postpartum Healing   120

THE HISTORY OF BIRTH IN THE UNITED STATES
by Dr. Stephanie Mitchell, "Doctor Midwife"   125

THE EMBODIMENTS:

AN INTRODUCTION TO THE COURT CARDS

PAGE OF CUPS   137

  EXERCISE: Ocean Visualization   138

PAGE OF SWORDS   141

PAGE OF WANDS   146

  TAROT SPREAD: Calling Sensual Command Into Your Birth Space   149

PAGE OF PENTACLES   151

  RECIPE: Bone Broth   154

EXERCISE: For Partners at Any Phase of Pregnancy,
Postpartum, or Parenting   157

RESOURCES FOR FURTHER EXPANSION   158

THE SOUL ARCHETYPES:
AN INTRODUCTION TO THE MAJOR ARCANA

0—THE FOOL   167

1—THE MAGICIAN   170

2—THE HIGH PRIESTESS   172

3—THE EMPRESS   175

4—THE EMPEROR   178
EXERCISE: Freewrite to Unearth Your Subconscious Biases About Birth   179

5—THE HIEROPHANT   182

6—THE LOVERS   184
EXERCISE: Write a Love Letter   185

7—THE CHARIOT   187

8—STRENGTH   189

9—THE HERMIT   191

10—THE WHEEL OF FORTUNE   194
JOURNAL: Breaking Generational Cycles   199

11—JUSTICE   200
TAROT SPREAD: Furthering Justice through Parenting   203

12—THE HANGED ONE   204

13—DEATH   206

14—TEMPERANCE   209

15—THE DEVIL   211

16—THE TOWER   214
EXERCISE: Comfort Measures for Moving through Intensity   219

CONTENTS

17—THE STAR   222

18—THE MOON   228

19—THE SUN   234

20—JUDGMENT   236

21—THE WORLD   239

CLOSING CEREMONY   243

Gratitude and Acknowledgments   245

To the parents who are ready to raise the generation

that will change the world.

—BMCH

To all the abuelas and birthing people in my family.

Our stories continue through your seeds.

Thank you for your wisdom and love.

—KR

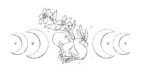

WELCOME

Welcome to *Tarot for Pregnancy*, a companion for radical, magical birthing folks. I'm elated that you have found your way to this book.

I am a full-spectrum doula, tarot reader, poet, photographer, mother, partner, aunt, and friend. I am of Scottish, Irish, Welsh, and American settler descent, and I grew up on unceded Anishinabewaki land in so-called Belleville, Michigan. My magical practice is rooted in both the attempt to heal and reckon with the harm of my more immediate ancestors, while also reaching back to the pre–Christian Inquisition pagan traditions of my more ancient ancestors. So, while this book may mention or refer to traditional practices from other Indigenous peoples, African diasporic cultures, East Asian Indigenous traditions, and so on, those are not cultures I belong to nor the lens through which I can teach. The tarot itself is not *only* a pagan European practice (as you will soon read, the "History of Tarot" chapter by Sanyu Estelle Nagenda delves deeper into this history for edification and clarification).

I am not a decades-long expert on either witchcraft or pregnancy and birth (at least not at the time of writing this book). If you were hoping for guidance from someone whose wisdom comes from an impressive number of years, put into this lifetime alone, then you'll likely be disappointed here. I am simply someone who is a voracious, insatiable student of birth, a witch finding her way back to what spirituality looked like for her ancestors before Christianity, and one who has a particular knack for connecting what the two topics of pregnancy and spirituality have to do with one another.

"I have a lot to learn. I have a lot to share."
—Chetna Mehta, creative wellness facilitator and artist*

....

* Find Chetna online at mosaiceyeunfolding.com and on social media @mosaiceye.

Since the first time I found out I was pregnant, the investigator in me was awakened. Even when I was just a pregnant person with no intentions of entering this field, I treated that experience like I was getting a PhD in pregnancy and birth—researching the root of things, and then the root of that root, and the root of that root and so on. To be clear, I do not have an actual PhD in anything.

In this book, you won't necessarily find a culmination of all that I've learned, because that type of scholarly literature is and has been led by Black birth workers* leading the reproductive justice† movement for decades. But I am constantly rooting my own work back into theirs, honoring how magic and pregnancy and birth intersect and intertwine, and how all can be enhanced by integration.‡

I want pregnant folks, or trying-to-become-pregnant folks, to consult this guide and be shaken by the shoulders with this message: Your intuition holds valid weight; it is powerful and should always be consulted when you make your choices during pregnancy and birth. I believe when tarot is used as a tool for introspection and spiritual connection, it has the ability to reignite your intuition's flame and can assist in deciphering what's "intuition" and what is fear-based thinking instilled by the overculture.

Tarot can be enlightening; it can be reassuring. And I want you to enjoy the process, but also, I want you to see where connecting to our ancient wisdom is the greatest gift we can give ourselves as pregnant, birthing beings.

I want pregnant folks or trying-to-become-pregnant folks to consult this guide and be confronted with another message, too—that choosing to have children is choosing to continue your ancestral legacy. Do you like what you'll be passing on? Are you even aware of what you'll be passing on? What do you need to heal or dismantle in yourself so that you aren't passing it on to the next generation?

Over the years of building a relationship with my tarot decks, I have learned that the cards are a proven confidant who will not bullshit you. Sometimes they are rude as hell and hurt your feelings. They can be a bitter, necessary medicine from your

....

* The works of Loretta Ross, Dorothy Parker, Chanel Porchia-Albert, Shafia Monroe, Racha Tahani Lawler, Margaret Charles Smith, and Stephanie Mitchell come to mind, to name a few.

† *Reproductive justice* is a term that marries reproductive rights and social justice defined by Loretta Ross as "a framework created by activist women of color to address how race, gender, class, ability, nationality, and sexuality intersect." It was first coined in 1994 by a group of Black women called Women of African Descent for Reproductive Justice.

‡ Honoring that in precolonial cultures, spirituality and birth were never separate, what I'm talking about in this book isn't revolutionary, it's remembering, for some reclaiming, and for others, like myself, repair.

guides who want what's best for your soul's growth, comfort be damned. Or the cards can be the bolstering, loving embrace of the ancestors who are proud of you. It is my firm belief that there is a place for both kinds of self-reflections in the movement toward improving birth outcomes in the United States.

I also want folks consulting this book to be routinely reminded of and rooted back into how magical and capable your body is, no matter your intersection* of abilities and identities. I am still going to argue that for you to be here reading this book, you and the vessel in which you plan to grow a human are magical. You are embarking on the alchemy of cell division. You are the magician alchemizing your creative fire, nutrients from the Earth, water, and your very breath into a new human.

Tell me that's not magic by its most basic definition.

Unfortunately, this world, as it is right now, will likely try to instill fear and self-doubt in you at some point in your journey. The white-supremacist, capitalist, ableist patriarchy is deeply woven into the foundational fabric of the medical industrial complex, where most pregnant people will birth in the United States. So, I hope that you'll let this guide be a continuous reminder of the truth of your magic, the validity of your intuition, and the innate dependability of your body's physiology.

....

* The concept of intersectionality was coined in 1989 by professor Kimberlé Crenshaw to describe how race, class, gender, and other individual characteristics "intersect," compounding oppressions and adding nuance to the experiences of folks who exist in identities that have been marginalized by the white-supremacist patriarchy.

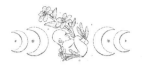

HOW TO USE THIS BOOK

This book is organized by Minor Arcana first, then the Embodiments (Court Cards), and then lastly the Soul Archetypes (the Major Arcana). This arrangement is because the aces through tens of the Minor Arcana correspond energetically and numerologically with the months of pregnancy from conception to birth, so I wanted them to be first for anyone reading along with their same month of pregnancy.

However, I advise reading the book in its entirety first, so you can know what's ahead and what to plan for, particularly in regard to birth. And then you can read the Minor Arcana one month at a time to know what's going on physically, energetically, and emotionally in the immediate moment, as in other pregnancy guides.

Then, of course, you can consult this book in readings you do for yourself to gain insight and clarity on your parenthood path. If you are a tarot reader who has a hard time interpreting the cards for pregnant people, I hope this guide is of service to you and the folks you serve.

The book itself can be used as a means of divination through the bibliomancy method of divination—meaning you can ground yourself, take a deep breath, close your eyes, and choose a page at random, trusting that it will hold the medicine needed for you in that moment.

You can also just read for your curiosity. I'm a believer that the things that interest you are the things *for* you, so if you jump around reading only what grabs your attention, trust that too.

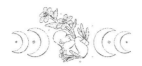

GLOSSARY OF TERMS

Below are terms and phrases that pertain to physiology, medical procedures, magic, tarot, culture, and more that you will find in this book or that I think you should know as a pregnant or planning-on-becoming-pregnant person. Each term or phrase is followed by a definition of what I personally mean when I use that term or phrase. However, I encourage further self-guided research on each topic that intrigues you.

adrenaline: the hormone emitted when fear is introduced and a fight-or-flight response is initiated, causing blood to rush to the arms and legs instead of to vital organs or to the baby.

anti-capitalism: recognition that the demands of keeping up with capitalism in order to obtain a secure livelihood are ableist, racist, sexist, and ageist; recognition that we should therefore be striving for a better way that works for and is safe for everyone, a way that doesn't equate our human worth with that of our productive value.

antiracism: "In a racist society, it is not enough to be non-racist, we must be antiracist." —Angela Y. Davis; a verb, a way of life that is in active, perpetual opposition of racism on a systemic and personal level.

archetype: a collectively inherited unconscious idea, pattern of thought, or image that is universally present, in individual psyches and represented in the Major Arcana of the tarot.

birth center: a true birth center is a space not affiliated with a hospital but may have a few more amenities than birthing at home. Access to medical interventions vary by birth center, but in general they do not perform surgical birth. At a birth center, births may be attended by both CNMs and/or CPMs.

bodyfeeding: feeding a baby from one's own body. A gender-inclusive term for breastfeeding or chestfeeding.

Cesarean birth: a surgical birth, the surgical removal of the baby through an incision in the abdomen. A nonemergency Cesarean will be done with just local epidural anesthesia while the birthing person is awake; an emergency Cesarean will likely be done under general anesthesia while the birthing person is asleep. It is rumored to go by this name because Julius Caesar was born this way, but like many aspects of Roman culture, much of their technologies were stolen from the continents they invaded and colonized, in this case Africa. Some of the earliest documentation of surgical birth was performed by Indigenous healers in Kahura, Uganda.

CNM: a certified nurse midwife, trained within the medical system as a nurse first and then given specialized training in labor and childbirth; usually attends births only at hospitals or hospital-affiliated birth centers; and are sometimes more open to utilizing modern/Western medicine interventions during birth, compared to traditional midwives, if the birthing person consents.

cortisol: the hormone produced when the body needs to respond to stress. There is some research showing that a cortisol signal from the baby to the pregnant person is what lets the body know that the baby is ready to be born and initiates the start of labor, which may be an explanation of why stress is a risk factor for preterm labor.

Court Cards: traditionally, these are the pages, knights, queens, and kings representing each suit, and their energy is easily connectable with embodied human archetypes, so for the purposes of this guide, I prefer to refer to them as "the Embodiments."

CPM: a certified professional midwife; usually attends births out of hospital at a birthing person's home or in a birth center. CPMs in many states are licensed to carry medicine and are more open to utilizing modern medicine methods during birth if the birthing person consents.

cultural appropriation: an arm of white supremacy wherein people with white-skin privilege take free license to borrow from and/or profit off cultural practices that are not their own; often cultural practices for which

white supremacy historically persecuted people of those cultures for practicing; contributes to the continued erasure of the original cultures those
practices were from. Cultural appropriation is highly present in the world
of birth work and spirituality in the form of widespread use of cultural practices such as Blessingway ceremonies held by non-Indigenous people, use
of rebozos during labor by people not of Mesoamerican descent, burning of
sage and palo santo by folks who are not of the Indigenous cultures in which
those plant medicines are ancestrally rooted, etc.

doula: a nonmedical professional companion throughout pregnancy and
birth who provides educational, emotional, and physical support to the
birthing person and advocates for the birthing person. (Note: Advocacy
might not necessarily be included in every doula's definition of what role a
doula should play, especially if they obtained their training through one of
the more formal programs available throughout the doula training industrial complex.)

free birth: planning and preparing for a birth at home without the atten-
dance of a midwife or any other kind of medical professional.

full-spectrum doula: a professional companion for all phases of the reproductive journey from abortion, pregnancy, miscarriage, stillbirth, birth,
and postpartum.

home birth: planning and preparing for a birth within your own home
attended by a CPM.

hospital birth: planning and preparing for leaving the home and going to
a hospital for labor and birth. I prefer to refer to this birthing place as an
"out-of-home" birth.

informed consent: permission granted in the full knowledge of the possible consequences, typically that which is given by a patient to a doctor for
treatment with full knowledge of the possible risks and benefits.

lunar energy: present in all humans regardless of gender identity or genitals; lunar energy is the part of us that is receptive, intuitive, empathetic,
wise, nurturing, and emotionally strong, grounded, creative. Lunar energy
is mysterious, fluid, and unknown. It is also the part of us that exercises

passive-aggressiveness or manipulation. (Note: Traditionally you'll see solar and lunar energy labeled as "masculine" and "feminine" energy respectively, which is a duality and balance or imbalance frequently referred to in the tarot. I choose not to use that language not only because of its adherence to the outdated gender binary and therefore inadvertent reinforcement of gender-based stereotypes, but also because the solar-lunar duality is more expansive and explanatory of the actual duality this language is trying to represent).

magic(k): exercising your influence over the subtle, invisible energies of the world; the etymology of the word *magic* has roots in the phrase "be able."

Major Arcana: twenty-two archetypes that make up the tarot, representing the universal, bigger-picture themes of life.

medical induction: the artificial starting of labor either manually by conducting a membrane sweep or by inserting a Foley balloon (inserted into the cervix, then inflated to slowly dilate the cervix), administering the drug Cervidil (dinoprostone) vaginally, or by the introduction of Pitocin (the artificial form of oxytocin administered through IV fluids).

medical-industrial complex: a term coined by Barbara and John Ehrenreich describing the network of corporations that supply health care services and products for a profit and the implications on the health care we receive in a for-profit health care system.

midwife: a medical professional educated and trained in normal physiologic birth, who is qualified to attend low-risk births. They are equipped with many medical resources in the event of interventions becoming necessary during a birth, but they are not equipped with all medical resources and are not qualified to perform surgical birth.

Minor Arcana: the cards of the tarot organized by four suits (wands, cups, swords, and pentacles), ace through ten. The energies of these archetypes represent the smaller-scale, everyday minutiae of life. For the purposes of this book, I align each Minor Arcana card with the correlating number of months along in pregnancy.

OB: an obstetrician, someone educated and trained in surgical birth, qualified to attend high-risk births, not trained in the hormonal or physical requirements of normal physiologic birth.

oxytocin: the hormone present when we feel good, comfortable, and happy; present in its most concentrated amounts during orgasm. The necessary hormone present in our bodies for the start and continuation of labor and birth, oxytocin regulates the intensity and frequency of contractions, and in unmedicated births it helps with coping with the pain of labor. Oxytocin is interrupted and sometimes halted by the hormone adrenaline. It is the necessary hormone for allowing a letdown of milk during bodyfeeding.

parenthood path/parenthood journey: refers to the whole spectrum of pregnancy, birth, postpartum, and parenting phases of life.

patriarchy: the assumption of cisgender men as dominant over women, trans folks, and nonbinary folks; a false but (consciously or subconsciously) widely accepted way of thinking that has reigned dominant for the past several centuries.

pregnant/birthing folks or pregnant person: inclusive terms that recognize and honor that not all people with uteruses who will become pregnant are women.

shadow work: the "shadow" is a concept introduced by psychologist Carl Jung referring to the unconscious or unseen parts of ourselves that influence our biases, actions, and decisions; shadow work takes steps or enacts practices to delve into your shadow and make the unconscious conscious so that you may heal any past traumas or conditioning that might be holding unwanted influence over you.

solar energy: present in *all* humans regardless of gender identity or genitals; solar energy is the part of us that exercises assertiveness, action, practicality, protectiveness, and physical strength. Solar energy is clear and obvious. It is also the part of us that exercises violence, unhealthy control, pride, and corruption. (Note: Traditionally you'll see solar and lunar energy labeled as "masculine" and "feminine" energy respectively, which is a duality and balance or imbalance frequently referred to in the tarot. I choose not to use that language not only because of its adherence to the outdated gender binary and therefore inadvertent reinforcement of gender-based stereotypes, but also because the solar-lunar duality is more expansive and explanatory of the actual duality this language is trying to represent.)

spell: a tangible way of practicing magic with the intention of influencing a certain outcome.

spiritual bypassing: a form of gaslighting wherein the offending person tries to side-step responsibility and reality by way of using spiritual ideas for dismissal of the offended person's lived experience (e.g., someone is accused of causing racist harm and they reply, "I'm not racist, I believe we're all one"). It also comes in the form of **toxic positivity** rampant in the spiritual world where a person is encouraged to remain incessantly positive despite the harsh realities of the world; avoids processing or dealing with anything difficult or "negative."

tarot: an ancient deck of cards depicting images of archetypes that apply to everyday experiences of life, often used for divination, self-reflection, or communication with ancestors, spirit guides, etc. Divided up into the Major arcana, the Minor arcana, and the Court Cards.

TOLAC/VBAC: trial of labor after Cesarean (TOLAC) is a planned or attempted vaginal birth after Cesarean (VBAC).

traditional midwife: attends births in an out-of-hospital setting and chooses not to utilize any medical advancements at all during prenatal care or birth, relying solely on the dependability of ancient technologies and trust of the body's physiological process during gestation and birth.

unmedicated birth: no drugs or medical interventions introduced during labor and birth at all.

vaginal birth: uterine contractions cause cervical dilation (widening) and effacement (softening and thinning), which makes way for the baby being born by being squeezed through the fully dilated cervix and vaginal canal through a series of cardinal movements. This helps express the fluid out of the baby's ears and causes the production of catecholamines. Dopamine, adrenaline, epinephrine, etc. are all catecholamines that occur in response to certain stressors; they are present in fetal lung fluid to promote lung maturation at the culmination of birth. Catecholamines are necessary for the reabsorption of fluid into the baby's lungs and responsible for the release of the surfactant that will line the baby's lungs once they have inflated after birth.

white supremacy: the assumption of whiteness as default; whiteness as nonracialized while everyone else is "other"; the assertion that people with white skin are smarter, better, or more advanced than people with any other skin color, but primarily most systemically and socially detrimental to people racialized as Black. White supremacy presents an imbalanced power dynamic to every aspect of our current overculture: health care of any kind, education, law enforcement, etc. A false but (consciously and subconsciously) widely accepted way of thinking that has reigned dominant for the past several centuries.

witch: someone who practices magic of any kind.

TAROT
FOR
PREGNANCY

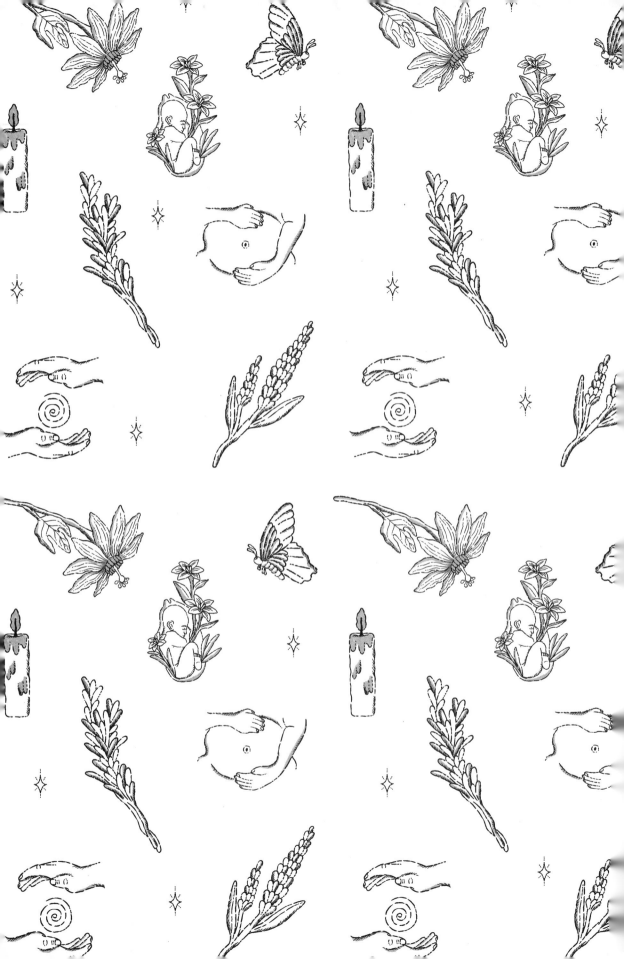

Too often we dive into adopting a spiritual practice before we even look into its cultural origins, understand its roots, or examine where we stand historically in relation with that practice. This can lead to appropriation of practices we culturally have no right to access or utilize, and it can also make us miss or ignore spiritual practices that *are* in alignment with our cultural heritage (and therefore more potent and useful for us specifically) simply because we aren't getting to the root of things to find them.

Knowing where any spiritual practice comes from is the first step in practicing it in right relationship, and when it comes to magic, integrity is everything. Tarot and cartomancy seems to be one of those spiritual practices that many different cultures historically had a hand in creating, and yet their history is still primarily told from the Anglo-European lens. Sanyu Estelle Nagenda offers the most in-depth compilation of all that was involved in the inception of cartomancy that I've personally ever come across.

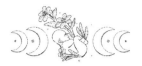

THE HISTORY [MYSTERY] OF TAROT

BY SANYU ESTELLE NAGENDA, "THE WORD WITCH"

There are many texts from over centuries, countries, and continents that speak to the history of the tarot, particularly from the time it cropped up in Europe in the 1400s. I will reiterate some of that information here, as well as offer insight into the etymology of the word *tarot* and *tarocchi*.

What I will add to this conversation is a more cohesive narrative of the lineage of the tarot itself—not from a mystical perspective, but rather from a geographical, cultural, and sociological perspective. Let us call it the mundane and mystical perspective, as the journey the tarot took to become what we appreciate it as now is quite a fool's journey all on its own.

The word, practice, game, and concept of *tarot* officially entered into the English language in the 1590s. It was adapted from French of the same spelling and translated from the Old Italian word *tarocchi*,* which itself came from the singular *toroccare*† and officially emerged (as the word we now associate with the divination tool) into the Italian language in the early 1500s.

Tarocchi cards emerged from somewhere within the regions of Milan, Ferrara,

---

* Ancient Italian card game also known as *minchiate* (a Florentine sister game to the tarot that came later) that preceded *picchetto*, which is a French invention. Tarot cards are usually finely painted, like miniatures on a gold-leaf background, dotted with specks forming graceful arabesque decorations and surrounded by a silver edge, in which the same dotted decorations depict a rotating spiral ribbon. Without a doubt this *tàra*, a print or impression made by tiny neatly aligned dots—compare Latin *taràre*, "to drill/pierce," similar to the classical *tèrere*, "to hit"—must have given tarot cards their name.

† Seems altered from *altercare* ("to argue") with *tarocco*, "to erupt with angry words; to argue/get upset; shouting loudly." This literal translation is a bit odd, but to me it can also be translated simply as "to play the tarot card game."

and Bologna, Italy (though they have been attributed as far as Florence), sometime in the 1420s. There is uncertainty as to whether tarot first emerged strictly as a card game or whether it was also initially used for divinatory readings.

That being said, the first known mentions of it are from legal documents that cite the complaints and testimony of friars and other clergymen from as early as 1450. Saint Bernardino of Siena said, "Various figures are painted . . . which figures show forth the mysteries of evil,"* while a Franciscan friar in Umbria preached a sermon stating, "There is nothing so hateful to God as the game of trumps [see page 14]. For everything that is base in the eyes of the Christian faith is seen in trumps."†

If this was simply a card game that was considered unchristian or licentious because of its relationship to gambling, I don't know that there would be so much focus on the figures outside of the Devil card, which incited much anger among clergymen. But it seemed commonly known, even among its antagonists, that there was something about tarot cards that wasn't of the same ordinance as the Christian faith.

Tarot cards were not the first cards to be banned by the papacy and the papal states. As playing cards were not indigenous to Europe, they made their way across the various provinces, states, and countries over century-long periods. Each country added something of its own to playing cards as well as inventing their own games and usage of the cards, which then made their way around Europe through travel and trade yet again.

What distinguishes tarot from playing cards is the addition of the Major Arcana, originally called "triumphs" cards before being shortened to "trumps" cards, as well as the option of the fourth Court Card within the Minor Arcana, originally called the suit cards, which typically consists of a page, knight, queen, and king. Originally playing cards had only three Court Cards and they were typically male figures: deputy, lieutenant, knight, or knave; second deputy, second lieutenant, jack, or squire; and king.

The first time playing cards were documented as being banned in Europe was almost one hundred years prior to the banning of tarot cards. In 1367 there was an injunction against gambling with playing cards in the Canton of Bern. This was followed by injunctions across Europe: Florence in 1376, Germany in 1378, Marseilles in 1381, and Paris and the city of Ulm, Germany, in 1397.

....

* Barbara G. Walker, *The Secrets of the Tarot: Origins, History, and Symbolism*. (New York: Harper & Row, 1984).

† Cynthia Giles, *The Tarot: History, Mystery and Lore* (New York: Atria Books, 1994).

The first two European countries to be introduced to playing cards were Spain and Italy. It was unclear where it was introduced first, but there are claims that the first words for playing cards came from Spanish, which itself came from Arabic, so there is reason to think Spain was made familiar with playing cards before Italy,* particularly as various proportions of Spain had been colonized by the Moors from 700 to 1600.

In the Levant—the lands east of the Mediterranean Sea—during the 600s, then called Arabia, the Prophet Muhammad died in 632. Right after this, the first caliphate ("the political-religious state comprising the Muslim community and the lands and peoples under its dominion in the centuries following the death of the Prophet Muhammad"†) took power.

From this point on, the Byzantine Empire northeast of the Levant called all people practicing Islam *Saracens*, which took in Northern Europe, whereas northwest of the Levant in the Mediterranean, the blanket term for practitioners of Islam became *Moors* (*blackamoors* and *white Moors*). There are, of course, many ethnic and cultural distinctions among the Muslims covered referred to by the terms *Saracen* and *Moor*.

The word *Moor* comes from the Latin word *Maurus* and was originally, literally, "inhabitant of Mauretania." Even the Latin was taken from the Greek *maurós*, which was a cognate for *black*. At the time, it was used to describe the Berbers and other African peoples from the ancient Roman colony of Mauretania in what is now Northern Algeria and Morocco. It came to be the blanket term for all the Muslims who ruled Spain, Europeans of African descent, and anybody who was darker skinned.

The word *Saracen* comes from the late Latin word *Saracenus*, which came from Greek *Sarakenos* and was itself taken from Arabic *sharquiyin* for "eastern" or "east."‡ However, during medieval times prior to the Renaissance, the name was associated with Sarah from the Bible. That is why the Byzantines as well as the Crusaders regularly referred to practitioners of Islam as Saracens.

The earliest reference to playing cards or dominoes, which are represented by the same character in Mandarin Chinese, is from tenth-century Chinese literature.

....

* Helen Farley, *A Cultural History of Tarot* (London: I. B. Taurus, 2009). https://stilluntitledproject.files .wordpress.com/2015/05/helen-farley-a-cultural-history-of-tarot-from-entertainment-to-esotericism -2009.pdf.

† Erin Blakemore, "Who Were the Moors?" *National Geographic*, December 12, 2019, https://www .nationalgeographic.com/history/article/who-were-moors.

‡ *Encyclopaedia Britannica Online*, s.v. "Saracen," accessed September 10, 2021, https://www.britannica .com/topic/Saracen.

There are no surviving descriptions of the game play or images of the game pieces.[*] The oldest surviving playing cards in the world date from between the eleventh and fifteenth century and are believed to come from al-Fustat,[†] the earliest Arab and Muslim settlement in Egypt as well as the site of the first mosque in Egypt.

Playing cards and the paper that allowed their construction made their way from China by way of the Silk Road, via boats and trade routes, through Africa Major, Asia Minor, the "Middle East," and the Southwest Asian/North African region. Within two centuries playing cards had traveled from China all the way to Egypt where the two oldest remaining playing cards in the world are from.

What is believed to be the oldest of these cards is the de Unger fragment(s) said to be from al-Fustat, and which are now items in the Keir Collection of Islamic Art. The second oldest remaining playing cards are the Mamluk cards said to be from the 1500s, which are located at the Topkapi Palace Museum in Istanbul.

Mamluk cards are the foundation of the playing cards we commonly use today in most anglophone cultures. They are also the foundation of the Minor Arcana within the tarot deck with only minor variation from its earliest known design. Mamluk cards are attributed to the Mamluk Sultanate, who ruled Egypt (and eventually Syria) between 1250 and 1517 before being overthrown by the Ottoman Empire.

While it is unclear if playing cards appeared first in Spain or Italy, what we do know is that playing cards made their way to Europe through Egypt, either through Spain or the Moors, who ruled various parts until the fall of Granada, or through the Mamluk Sultanate, who established vigilantly watched trade routes with various European rulers including the Andalusian Muslims of what we today call Spain.

What seems clear is that regardless of however long the Muslim world was playing cards, they did not produce or share the playing cards that became the predecessor of today's card games with Europe until the Mamluk Sultante had been in power for at least one hundred years. Once the Mamluk cards spread across Europe, all other European card derivations came from it.

So, who were the Mamluks and why were they so influential? The answer is complex and deeply steeped in crosscultural relations. Ultimately, the Mamluks were a special caste of peoples within Muslim states who had been a staple and designated class of the enslaved since the rise of the first caliphate. Back then the

....

[*] Robert M. Place, *The Fool's Journey: The History, Art, & Symbolism of the Tarot* (Saugerties, NY: Talarius, 2010).

[†] J. Jordan, *Islamic Playing Card Fragments in the Keir Collection at the Dallas Museum of Art.*

first Muslims formed the caliphate and spread the practice of Islam through con-
quest.

The word *Mamluk* itself means "owned" in Arabic and has long been used to describe the peoples that were most desired as enslaved peoples by the various Sunni
Muslim states of the time, first called caliphates and then, eventually, sultanates.
These enslaved peoples were primarily from the Black Sea region, namely the Balkans, the former state of Circassia, as well as around the Caspian Sea.

By the time this enslavement route was well underway, most people who were
enslaved were of Kipchak Turkic origin, with a second large wave of the enslaved peoples being specifically of Circassian heritage from at least the mid-fourteenth century
onward because the Kipchak Turks had basically been enslaved into extinction.[*]

Turkic peoples of this time and these regions were sometimes Muslim, often
pagan, not culturally and linguistically Arab, and even when they were Muslim not
necessarily the same sect of Muslim (which at the time were Sunni). Regardless, the
enslaved were always converted to the faiths and practices of their enslavers as well
as trained in the roles they were purchased to hold.

During the eleventh through about the sixteenth century, it seems both Muslim
and European people of means preferred servants and enslaved people of lighter
skin for different reasons. In the caliphates and sultanates, it was because of the
value of the people from the aforementioned regions as both trained soldiers and for
harems, whereas in Europe there was always attention on pigmentation down to the
differentiation between "blackamoors" and "white Moors" even though among
themselves the Moors shared a faith and had their own caste system that ranked
their demographics differently.

During medieval times in Europe, many indentured peoples came from Europe's
own native peasantry. There were laws within the Byzantine Empire and the caliphates
that natives of their regions could not be enslaved. So, while Western and Central Europeans could call upon their own populace to do servant work, the Byzantine Empire
and the caliphates had to source their enslaved populations from outside their own
citizenry. In the Byzantine Empire, that meant Muslims, "pagans" (peoples who were
not Catholic or Jewish) from Eastern Europe, and Africans who practiced indigenous
traditions that weren't Judaism, Christianity, or Islam. For the caliphates that meant
Catholics, pagans from Eastern Europe, non-Arab Africans who practiced indigenous

....

[*] "Egypt, 1000–1400 A.D.," in *Heilbrunn Timeline of Art History* (New York: The Metropolitan Museum of
Art, 2000). http://www.metmuseum.org/toah/ht/?period=07&region=afe (October 2001).

traditions that weren't Judaism, Christianity, or Islam, and even some minority Muslim groups from outside the caliphate such as from the Balkans.

Western Europe, being in the middle of all this trading and playing both sides, carried out an enslavement trade of demand in addition to pulling their own servants from their native peasant populations. They played both the Byzantine Empire and the Caliphate to great effect:

> The trade routes of African slaves ran from the sub-Sahara and East Africa to the Mediterranean South (trans-Saharan routes) and Near East (via the Persian Gulf); and of European slaves from Northeastern Europe to the Byzantine-Arab Mediterranean. The latter were called (in the Arabic of Andalusia) *saqaliba*, referring to their Slavic origin.*

All this is to say that enslavement was alive and well around the Mediterranean and during medieval times. This was true of all three powers that ran that region during the medieval period: Latinized Europe, the Byzantine Empire, and the caliphates. It just so happens that both the Almohad and Ayyubid Dynasties preferred to enslave the Kipchak/Qipchaq peoples and Turkic people in general. This practice increased during the Crusades when the Almohad Empire spanned the whole of North Africa including Moorish Spain (as the Berber Muslim Empire), up until the middle of the thirteenth century. This did not include Egypt, which was run by the Ayyubid Sultanate (the Sunni Muslim Empire), which started with the reign of Kurdish General Saladin, who ruled Egypt from 1169 until the death of Al-Malik al-Ṣāliḥ Ayyūb in 1249.

During the Ayyubid Sultanate's rule of Egypt, every general from Saladin included the practice of importing Mamluk slaves and training them as soldiers who then made up the sultanate's private armies. They provided them with forces that were not just religiously tied to their power like the militaries of all sultanates but also socially and economically invested in the success of Egypt, which protected and gave high status to the Mamluk. All Mamluk peoples did go through conversions to Islam, but their primary tutelage was in matters of state and of war, and they quickly

---

* Anastasius Philoponus, "Medieval Mediterranean Slave Trade—Slaves in the Eastern Roman ('Byzantine') World," Novo Scriptorium, September 25, 2019, https://novoscriptorium.com/2019/09/25/medieval-mediterranean-slave-trade-slaves-in-the-easter-roman-byzantine-world/.

rose in rank within the sultanate's power system because they were so essential to the independence of Egypt during the Crusades.[*]

In 1249 Al-Malik al-Ṣāliḥ Ayyūb became gravely ill during a Crusades campaign and had to retreat into hiding. He died, but his Mamluk generals, soldiers, and wife devised a scheme so that nobody was aware of this. Unlike the Berber, Sunni, or Arab sultanates before them, the Mamluk did not pass down power through lineage or race. They gave rank to their most powerful members regardless of their class, lineage, or ethnicity. After Al-Malik al-Ṣāliḥ Ayyūb's death, his widow, Shajar al-Durr, was placed on the throne as the first and only woman sultan. This marked the end of the Ayyubid Sultanate and began the era of Mamluk rulership of Egypt.

There is evidence of European versions of Mamluk cards as early as 1367, and these cards had to travel far and wide enough to be used among all classes as well as become noticed by clergymen in multiple countries. Additionally, the oldest surviving playing cards that we know of are thought to have been found in al-Fostat in Egypt.

So, it is safe to assume that it was under the Egyptian Mamluk Sultanate and the climate created by them that Mamluk Cards started to be produced in earnest. They were not traditional leaders, and they made that clear by backing a woman sultan at what was arguably the most perilous time in establishing their rulership. This differentiates them from the Circassian Mamluk Sultanate:

> There is universal agreement among historians that the Mamluk state reached its height under the Turkish sultans and then fell into a prolonged phase of decline under the Circassians. The principal achievements of the Turkish Mamluks lay in their expulsion of the remaining crusaders from the Levant and their rout of the Mongols in Palestine and Syria; they thereby earned the thanks of all Muslims for saving Arabic-Islamic civilization from destruction. It is doubtful, however, that such a goal figured in their plans; rather, as rulers of Egypt they were seeking to reconstitute the Egyptian Empire.[†]

By 1250 the Mamluk Sultanate had formally seized power, attempted to put a woman sultan on the throne who they could rule alongside, expelled all Crusaders

---

[*] Suzan Yalman, "The Art of the Mamluk Period (1250–1517)," October 2001, Metmuseum.org. Retrieved September 10, 2021, from https://www.metmuseum.org/toah/hd/maml/hd_maml.htm.

[†] *Encyclopaedia Britannica Online*, s.v. "Mamluk," https://www.britannica.com/topic/Mamluk.

from the entire Levant by mobilizing Mamluks of other sultanates, *and* sustained control of all Egypt and its port cities at the same period that the Mamluk cards not only emerged but spread.

Whether it was Mamluk sultan(s), generals, or traders who allowed Mamluk cards to be brought to Europe's attention is unclear. What is known is that it was through nobility playing card games that their popularity spread and playing card games became common. At that time paper was expensive and playing cards were hand painted. This wouldn't be something in the possession of someone who didn't have some wealth or status, or who was not the creator of the cards.

Because the Mamluk Sultanate had successfully banned all Crusaders from the Levant, it was extremely taxing and dangerous for European people who were not traders or nobility to travel throughout the Muslim world. Europeans were uniformly discriminated against in court proceedings, traders were only sanctioned to visit certain trading posts, and nobility were on ever-shifting terms with both the caliphates and the sultanates.[*]

It seems very unlikely that it was the Crusaders who were responsible for bringing back playing cards at the rate it would take for playing cards to spread among nobility and become popular across all Europe. They were busy killing followers of Islam while also attempting to avoid being killed at every turn. That seems like a full-time job that doesn't exactly allow for large-scale distribution of a foreign game played by Muslims.

That being acknowledged, once these cards made their way from Egypt across the Mediterranean sometime in the late 1200s, they quickly spread across Europe. Whether first through Spain or Italy, playing cards were probably brought by the Moors and/or through high-ranking generals, artisans, or traders from Egypt and other Muslim port cities. Perhaps nobility from the sultanates or Europe might also be responsible.

It is unclear how popular these games were among Muslim citizenry of the many sultanates, but as there are not a great deal of (popularly known or accessible) references to these cards in those regions at this time, nor many surviving specimens of these cards, it isn't unwarranted to assume they were a pastime of the upper classes for at least a century.

Once these Mamluk cards changed cultures, they also changed in format. The nature of card games and playing cards transformed from border to border and

....

[*] F. Apellániz, "Chapter 1 Introduction," in *Breaching the Bronze Wall* (Leiden, The Netherlands: Brill, 2020) doi: https://doi.org/10.1163/9789004431737_002.

country to country depending on what was relevant to the culture at the time. Regardless of being side by side, Spain, Italy, France, and Germany all changed the suits of their playing cards to better fit their preferences. Similarly, imagery that was not allowed under Muslim law was added to playing cards in Europe.[*] Whereas in the original Mamluk cards there were only symbols, numbers, and titles, once playing cards reached Europe, queens (originally in German and French decks) and pages (originally women in French and Italian decks) were added to the standard playing card deck. This is how the Court Cards became four instead of three.

Originally the Mamluk deck consisted of four suits: scimitars, coins, cups, and polo sticks.[†] Within each of these suits there were ten numbered cards and three royal cards. In the Mamluk deck, those Court Cards were governors/kings, upper marshal/lieutenants (who became queens) and lower marshal/second lieutenants (who became knights, knaves, or pages depending on the region).

When playing cards became standardized in Italy—which I will focus on because that is where tarot cards emerged—they stopped substituting the queen for the lieutenant and just gave her a card of her own, thereby cementing the four–Court Card deck as a standard option of play even as three–Court Card decks remained. They also started drawing the Court Card images instead of just listing them as "King" or "Queen." Italy then replaced the actual lieutenant card with the knight and alternated between making the second lieutenant either the Knave or the Page. As far as the suits go, they largely remained the same as the Mamluk deck, simply substituting swords for scimitars and batons for polo sticks. In Europe, the game of polo was not yet known, so Italians of the 1300s had to change the suit to something more relatable and commonly spoken of.

With the advancement of technology, playing cards became easier to manufacture. Stencils and stamps took over work originally made only by painters and artists. This allowed playing cards to trickle down from the nobility to the merchant and peasant populations, where it was both noticed and increasingly unappreciated by Roman Catholic clergymen as well as local religious institutions.

Thus, there were lawful complaints from as early as 1367 all the way through to 1450, at which point we know the tarot had already mysteriously emerged. The origins of this deck do seem to want to remain a mystery. As stated earlier, the

. . . .

[*] P. Huson, *Mystical Origins of the Tarot: From Ancient Roots to Modern Usage* (United States: Inner Traditions/Bear, 2004).

[†] T. Gjerde, *Historical Playing Cards*. Mamluk cards, ca. 1500. https://cards.old.no/

birthplace of tarot is thought to be somewhere between Milan, Ferrara, and Bologna, even while Florence is still claiming to be its potential birthing place.

The unknown Franciscan friar referred to at the beginning of this chapter was in Umbria when he spoke on the *utilis de ludo*—the use of games. Umbria is not far from Ferrara, Bologna, or Florence, and so it seems likely that he was exposed regularly and regionally to what he then referred to as "the triumphs" (later "trumps"), which were considered to be a different game from just cards.*

By the early 1500s the "triumphs," originally *trionfi* in Italian and later "the trumps" in English, were known as a twenty-two-picture card game that suddenly appeared in Central Italy. Originally intended to join the fifty-two or fifty-six suit cards as triumphs intended to "best" the other four suits in play, eventually the trumps were also played without the suit decks.

There are many, many books on how the original game of tarot was played as well as how both tarot and playing cards might have been used for divination, council, and as a means of observation from the very beginning of tarot's emergence forward. I will not be going there in this chapter as that ground is well tread upon, but I'll leave us with this.

When the triumphs cropped up in the early 1400s to combine with standard Italian playing cards and—together—create the tarot deck, most of the deck had already been through a long and fairly well documented journey.

While it is the Major Arcana, or the twenty-two trump cards, that distinguish a tarot deck from an Oracle deck or a deck of playing cards, the Minor Arcana are the majority of the tarot deck numbering fifty-six cards in total. That is 72 percent of the tarot deck. The Major Arcana certainly carries a lot of significance in esoteric and spiritual communities that practice tarot, but they are not more telling than the Minor Arcana when it comes to reading the cards and divining what is going on in your life or the life of friends, family, or clients. If a client gets all swords, wands, cups, and pentacles when being read by a tarot deck, that reading is no less a tarot reading simply because there are no Major Arcana involved. The Major and Minor Arcanas complete a system of observation, and both are necessary in the support of the other.

I find it fascinating that even though infinitely little is known about the Major Arcana and who brought them to the consciousness of Italians—before capturing the

....

* C. Giles, *The Tarot: History, Mystery and Lore* (Norway: Atria Books, 1994).

imagination of the French and the British (who added their own flourishes)—as a foundational twenty-two-card suit, so much more is known and documented about the Minor Arcana when one just goes back and does the digging. I would argue the lineages of the suit cards themselves boast all the qualities of the suit themes: swords (mind/air/relationship with self), cups (emotions/water/relationship with other), wands (personality/fire/relationship with groups), and pentacles (body/earth/relationship with environments).

The archetypes that became popularized as a result of the spreading of tarot are also very interesting. For instance, the card (un)popularly known as "The Tower" actually began its journey in the Major Arcana as "The Arrow"; later becoming "The House of God" before settling on its modern moniker. Similarly, "The Pope" and "The Popess" became "The Hierophant" and "The High Priestess," but, for a time, "The Popess" was removed because of outrage that she (and women in general) should be given position equivalent to the Pope (and a man)* in imagery or in practice.

So even the little we know about the arrival of the Major Arcana still lends itself to the lineage of having to go on one's own (though theirs was smaller and more regional—to Europe) fool's journey. Together, the triumphs/trumps and the suits or the Major and the Minor Arcana depict, relay, and foresee the journey of "The Fool."

As individuals who choose to divine with the tarot deck—which is really just a different form of play (so they're still playing cards!)—we are all dealt "the same hand" in that everyone is given the entire spectrum of the journey. All seventy-eight cards are in the possession of the reader or the client at the outset of a tarot session!

Before the cards are dealt anything can happen. Once the cards have been pulled from the deck, that's the order of the relevant narrative. We all start as the Fool in tarot. After that, anybody's shuffle can say. Some of us may go from the Fool to the suit of cups; some of us from the Fool to the World; but we will all go on the Fool's journey. The Fool is the "ground zero" of existential or human experience. From the position of the Fool, the rest is still unwritten and the mystery still unknown. Until it is uncovered, turned over, or discovered through osmosis. That is the medicine of the upright Fool: learning through osmosis. Having no worry about the past and no anxiety about the future because they give everything they have to the present moment, which is the only moment they pay attention to.

....

* H. Farley, *A Cultural History of Tarot* (New York: IB Tauris & Co Ltd, 2009). Retrieved September 10, 2021, from https://stilluntitledproject.files.wordpress.com/2015/05/helen-farley-a-cultural-history-of-tarot-from-entertainment-to-esotericism-2009.pdf.

I can only imagine what parts of the lineage of this practice we can put together when we have cross-cultural ties that allow for the research and translation of all the documents that must still remain in some government box, or some national archive, or even some little private corner of the internet. If my journey has inspired you to further this learning, I strongly encourage you to take the baton and move forward from here.

Sanyu Estelle is a Claircognizant ("clear knowing") Soothsayer ("truth teller") who is also known as "The Word Witch" because of her deep love for word origins (etymology) and word culture (philology). These natural inclinations are bolstered by an eleven-plus-year practice of Taoism that began with three years of training in Qi Gong and Tai Chi with Master Zi of Dharma Health Institute; as well as a ten-plus-year relationship with Ifa, the indigenous tradition of the Yoruba people of now-Nigeria, culminating in membership at Ile Orunmila Afedefeyo in Los Angeles led by Baba Fasegun and his daughter Iya Fayomi.

Sanyu identifies as a pigmented (82 percent), womoonist (as constant as the tides; word to Alice Walker), cissy (femme and fem), flexible asexual (it's a spectrum, seems unwise to call it), travel-apt (Earth is a country), and fashion-forward (Funk Flag Flyage) SSJW (sarcastic social justice warrior).

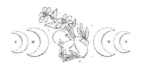

A NOTE ON REVERSALS

AND WHAT IT MEANS TO HAVE
A CONVERSATION AND RELATIONSHIP
WITH YOUR TAROT CARDS

A "reversal" is when a card appears upside down in a spread or a one-card pull. Whether or not to read into a card coming up as reversed is sometimes a point of controversy in the tarot-reading community.

Some folks and many traditional tarot guidebooks will say that a reversal indicates the exact inverse of the card's meaning, or that card's "negative" side. In a rejection of that archaic thought, some tarot readers will ignore reversals entirely, because to read all reversals as an inverse of their upright meaning would result in an imbalanced amount of "negativity" possible in any given reading. Sometimes folks who believe the latter will go so far as to turn all the cards upright.

One thing is certain to me: Reversals mean something, and while, no, they don't just mean the bad version of that card, they shouldn't be righted or ignored either. Here are some of the ways I read reversals, which are different for every reading:

- In a one-card pull or when using an oracle deck, you are asking for a complete sentence. But in a full tarot spread, you're engaging in a conversation with the cards, Spirit, your ancestors, or your subconscious (whatever aligns with your beliefs), a conversation that meanders, has tangents, *buts*, *ifs*, and *maybes*. In this way, to ignore a reversal is to erase one of the methods of language available with the cards. Sometimes a reversal will act as a question mark—you ask your cards, *How can I better connect with my intuition?* and a High Priestess reversed might throw that question right back at you: *What makes you think you are disconnected from it in the first place?* Often, reversals can indicate a *"but..."* For example: High Priestess (meaning get quiet and listen to your intuition) + Page of Wands reversed (but!) + Emperor (ground your actions in practical reality too, not just the whimsy of the Page, or the esoterism of the High Priestess). If that sounds too complicated, know that reading tarot is like learning any other language; it takes time and practice to understand. It's also a language where what you *feel* holds actual meaning.

- Sometimes a reversal is simply trying to draw your attention to that card's energy. Anything that disrupts the normal in a reading (or in general really) tends to capture our attention more than the cards that look "right," so in this case, a reversal can simply be yelling, *Hey! Look at me!*

- A reversal can indicate an obstacle or a blockage in a card's energy in your life, or sometimes even a refusal to allow its energy to enter into your life. This can be particularly true in spreads where one card indicates you, and another card indicates your goals, but a reversal stands visually between them—the reversed card can indicate what's in the way of what you're trying to achieve. For example, the Hanged One reversed ends up looking upright in most decks, which can indicate either a resistance to the surrender that the Hanged One asks for or a blockage preventing you from feeling safe enough to surrender.

- On that note, I am an advocate for spreads because then you can pay attention to how cards look in relation to one another in the conversation that is your tarot spread. In this way, sometimes a reversal can merely be trying to visually point to another card in the spread, such as an Ace of Cups reversed positioned over the Three of Cups upright indicating pouring your emotional energy into watering your community and close circle of soul kin. In general, reversed or not, pay attention to what card the swords are aiming at, where the wands are pointing, or what the cups are pouring into. All this holds meaning in your conversation with the cards.

- Lastly (not because these are the only ways to read reversals, but because these are the only ways I plan to discuss them), a reversal can indicate that you are already complete with something or ready to release it.* I find this to be a likely option if the last card you pull in a

....

* The concept or option of reading a reversal as a "completion" is a concept I learned from tarot teacher Lindsay Mack in their podcast *Tarot for the Wild Soul* (see Resources, page 158) and a series of three episodes where they talked about reversals specifically.

spread ends up being reversed. In that case, you can probably release that energy, or maybe you already have. But ultimately only you will know if a card is reversed because you are complete with its energy, which is why how you feel when a reversal comes up is so important.

On that note, pay attention to how you feel when a reversal appears because there are multitudes of ways to read reversals. Are you triggered by the sight of it and experiencing a nervous system response? Probably something to pay attention to there. Are you indifferent to the sight of that reversal? Probably something you've already released, or the reversal is just pointing to another card in the spread.

So how will you know which way to read yours? The answer is feeling, trusting, and being brave. Feel—what's your instinct for what this reversal means? Trust—trust that your feelings are valid. Be brave—this means not choosing the easiest way to read a card just to avoid accountability. Being brave and honest with yourself is a necessary ingredient for anyone reading tarot for themselves. Depending on what you believe, when you consult a tarot deck, it is your ancestors on the other end of the phone line. Expect the loving but firm counsel of your favorite auntie or sage great-grandpa. Deep down we know when we're avoiding a hard thing just because accountability is hard or change is hard. When it feels like there's two ways to read a card and one way calls you to accountability, while the other way isn't challenging to you in any way, it's usually more enlightening to explore the one that feels challenging.

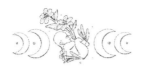

A NOTE ON REPEATING CARDS

Repeating cards occur when you are giving yourself a tarot reading from more than one deck and the same archetype appears more than once. Or if you pull multiple cards, but don't lay them down in a spread and instead keep shuffling, and the same card appears more than once. Or when you do multiple readings for yourself over time and the same card continuously appears.

Thanks to the brilliance and accuracy of AAVE,* there is a perfect explanation for repeating cards: It is a divine *I said what I said*. As in, sometimes the cards already gave you their answer, but we keep asking because we're hoping for more spelled-out clarity or obvious instruction. Or maybe because we're hoping for another answer than what we got. Either way, you undoubtedly got your answer.

If this happens for you in a reading, give thanks. In the magical occult world, moments of complete and absolute clarity are rare. In fact, acceptance of mystery, uncertainty, and the unknown are generally necessary fires to walk through when we engage in magic. The cards repeating themselves is highly unlikely statistically, so you know that a repeating card is ancestrally intentional. Even if it doesn't make sense to you in the moment, hold on to that message and wait for when you realize its applicability to your life. The time will always come if you allow for it.

....

* *AAVE* stands for "African American Vernacular English," and it refers to the language and colloquial phrases used by the Black community in the so-called United States, that often gets appropriated and then absorbed into the popular culture vernacular.

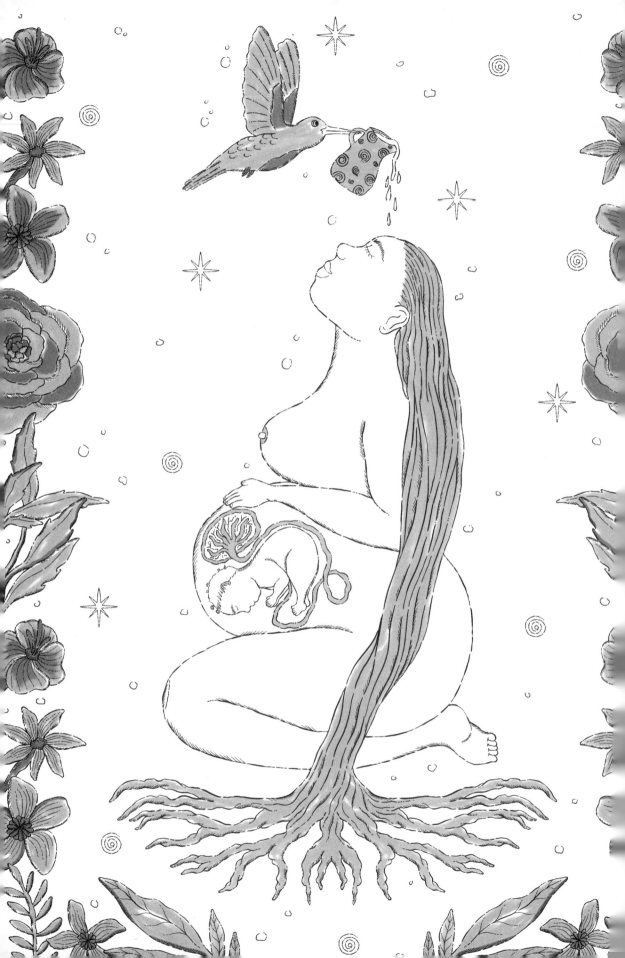

THE MINOR ARCANA

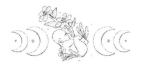

THE MINOR ARCANA

CONCEPTION–BIRTH

The divine realization that the energy of each number of the Minor Arcana aligns poignantly with the energy of each month of pregnancy was one of the major catalysts that inspired me to write this book. The energy of the Aces speaks directly to the experiences of fertility, conception, and those very first early weeks of finding out you're pregnant. The energy of the Fives speak directly to the intensity of transitions that occur when you're in your fifth month of pregnancy, the halfway point when things start feeling real and birth is no longer a distant prospect. The energy of the Tens happens to align perfectly with the myriad of experiences that come in the final weeks of pregnancy, birth, and then early postpartum. I've also found this to be true for every number in between, both personally and in my anecdotal research.

Traditionally, the energies of the Minor Arcana cards represent the minutiae of daily life, whereas the Majors address or represent the bigger life lessons, meanings, or transitions. So, it could be said that the Minors deal with the earthly realm—the body and mind—while the Majors deal with the spiritual realm—the soul.

Through the Minor Arcana, you will find a brief description of what's going on in your physical body for each month of pregnancy, such as the growth of your fetus, possible symptoms you're experiencing, and so on. These sections will be labeled "In the physical body" and they won't be quite as exhaustive as a full pregnancy guide like *Nurture* by Erica Chidi Cohen, or *Mama Glow* by Latham Thomas. The purpose of these sections is to continuously connect the growth, symptoms, or transitions back to the metaphysical explanation I'll be giving for each individual card, to help you see for yourself just how connected they are.

You can read these chapters in tandem with the month that you're currently experiencing in your pregnancy, or you can of course consult this book as you would any other tarot guide—reading a card's meaning as it shows up in your own tarot readings. There will be some suggested tarot spreads, journaling prompts, and helpful herbal recipes all intended to accompany certain points in your pregnancy.

I hope you can feel my genuine support, care, and blessings infused into every word of this book. And I hope you feel that energy accompanying you on this magical, expansive journey.

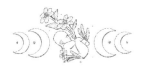

THE ACES

Look [at the ripples]. . . . So small at first, then look how they
grow. But someone has to start them.

—Grandmother Willow, *Pocahontas*

⊰ MONTH 1 THEMES ⊱

*conception, creation, implantation, a seed, a gift, an idea, inspiration,
the start of the journey, realizations, clarity of truth*

IN THE PHYSICAL BODY

Your estimated due date is calculated from the first day of your last menstrual cycle even though we know that the shedding of the uterine lining, the follicular phase, ovulation, fertilization, and implantation all still have to occur before you're actually "pregnant" (over the period of about two weeks). So, in this way, when we say you're "four weeks pregnant," your body has been building up to being pregnant for about two weeks, and you've only had a fertilized implanted egg for two weeks.

It's not unusual to not even know you're pregnant yet at this stage in pregnancy. While there can be some spotting or discomfort during implantation, you might not be feeling symptomatic of pregnancy until the progesterone hormone starts ramping up to try to hold on to the implanted egg. It might even be too early to test positive on a pregnancy test, but when you do test positive, that test is picking up on the hormone hCG (human chorionic gonadotropin). When your body does begin to produce higher amounts of hCG, that hormone is responsible for continuing the production of progesterone (to prevent uterine contractions so the fertilized egg can implant) and estrogen (allowing your uterus to stretch, increasing blood flow, and already preparing the milk ducts in breast/chest tissue). It is this hormone combination that is responsible for any nausea you may feel, intense moods, bloating, or sensitivities.

A note on progesterone: If you have a history of miscarriage, then you may want to consider the use of a topical progesterone cream to help your body hang on to the fertilized egg. While there are some physical side effects, it is widely accepted to be safe. Consult with your midwife or doctor about the use of progesterone, keeping in mind that most OBs do not consider miscarriages to be concerning until they've occurred multiple times in a row.

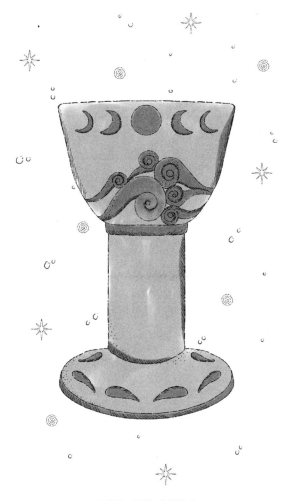

ACE OF CUPS

You are being given the gift of an emotional journey, and you are just at the beginning of it. Typically, Aces are seen as good omens, and this one is no exception. But know that when you are at the start of a journey, everything is still ahead of you—the joys and successes, frustrations and pains.

The work here is to not shy away from allowing yourself to feel. Your tears are information. How your body activates, vibrates, tingles, itches, and feels in different places when you interact with certain people or when you get exciting or triggering news—that's also information. Don't cover up emotion, or you'll miss the gift of the Ace of Cups.

Mitigating anxiety is likely going to be a common theme during your first month of pregnancy, but try to seek out methods of coping that don't bypass any difficult emotions you may be experiencing. Now is a good time to take stock of what methods of bolstering emotional well-being are accessible to you, whether that's meditation, therapy, journaling, aromatherapy, breath work, words of affirmation, nutritious movement, and so on—not all these modalities will be accessible to every pregnant person, but I'm sure at least one of them can be. And now is a great time to start solidifying a practice that allows you to integrate difficult emotions and mitigate stress instead of stuffing them down only to resurface later.

The Ace of Cups is our introduction to the element of water, the suit of how our emotional body communicates. Sometimes that's a raging sea, and sometimes that's a placid lake, and every bubbly, meandering stream in between.

For the next nine months, your baby-to-be is going to be an aquatic being, until their birthday when their instincts instruct them to pull in air to inflate their lungs for the first time and they become land mammals. Until then they'll be in a body of water called amniotic fluid, and eventually they'll practice moving that fluid in and out of their lungs and gulping. So, please, stay hydrated! You can calculate how much water you specifically should be drinking by taking your body weight, dividing that number in half, and then drinking that many ounces of water per day. In the later months of pregnancy, if you're having issues with low amniotic fluid or premature rupture of membranes, know that you can replenish your own fluids.

Water is their entire environment, which makes your own emotions a potent communicator at this time. Before they've even developed ears to hear your words, your baby can feel what you feel.

So, when you feel an intense fear, a sudden rush of adrenaline from getting cut off in traffic, anxiety about XYZ first thing when you wake up, frustration or anger over the state of the world, remember to also communicate feelings of joy, pleasure, and peace. Keep your growing baby in the loop over the next nine months. When you're feeling an intense emotion, explain why, and reassure them of their safety and yours.

Some babies who are destined to be healers might take your repeated experiences of danger as a sign that you need them earthside sooner than later. Though chronic stress is a proven cause of preterm labor with its own scientific reasons, this is a spiritual perspective on *why* exactly stress can cause preterm labor: your baby might think you need them.

So, anything that activates your nervous system—tough conversations with your care provider, a fight with your partner, a close call in traffic, the daily racial weathering that it is to live in a body that has been marginalized by white supremacy—reduce your exposure to that which poisons your peace, as much as you are able. *And* because upsetting events are inevitable and I don't want the fact that you're experiencing distress while pregnant to cause even *more* stress, remember to communicate another emotional story to your baby too. You can do this by taking deep intentional breaths into your belly, setting aside time to meditate and connect with your baby, enjoying a favorite meal, laughing, masturbating, or spending time in the community that makes you feel loved and held.

ꙮ ACE OF CUPS THEMES ꙮ

beginnings, the element of water, heart chakra, emotions overflowing, emotions as communicators, stress management, expanding your capacity for love

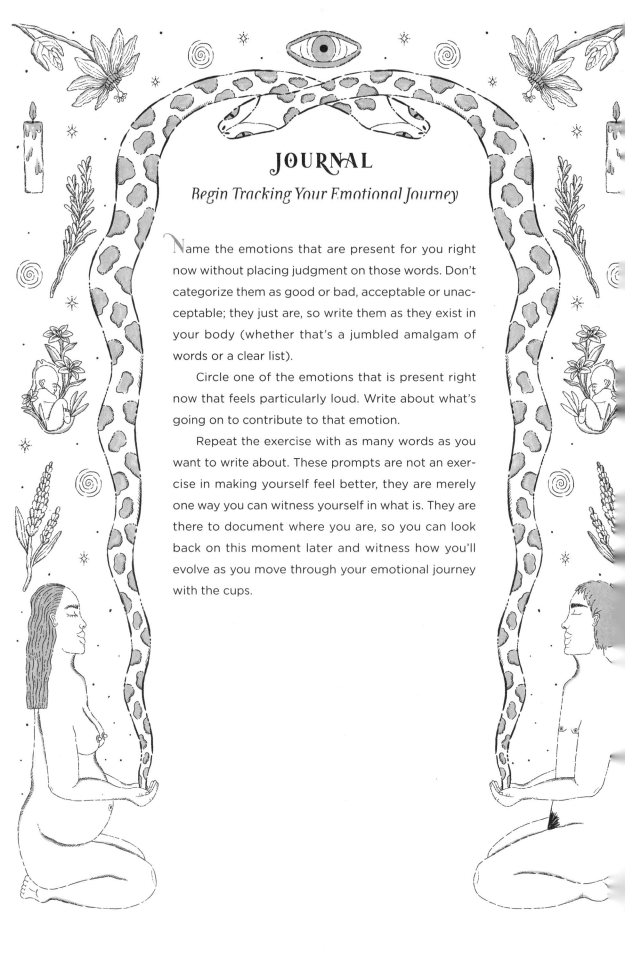

JOURNAL

Begin Tracking Your Emotional Journey

Name the emotions that are present for you right now without placing judgment on those words. Don't categorize them as good or bad, acceptable or unacceptable; they just are, so write them as they exist in your body (whether that's a jumbled amalgam of words or a clear list).

Circle one of the emotions that is present right now that feels particularly loud. Write about what's going on to contribute to that emotion.

Repeat the exercise with as many words as you want to write about. These prompts are not an exercise in making yourself feel better, they are merely one way you can witness yourself in what is. They are there to document where you are, so you can look back on this moment later and witness how you'll evolve as you move through your emotional journey with the cups.

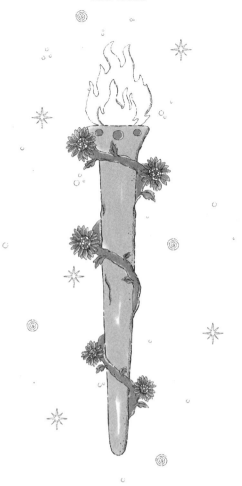

ACE OF WANDS

"Creation begins with desire."

—Paige Hasaballah, visual creator*

You are being given the gift of a creative journey, and you are setting out on it with purpose and intention.

Though it's not often thought of this way, pregnancy is one of the ultimate expressions of creativity. Your body is the artist, making a masterpiece of cell division. Your body is an alchemist—taking a very specific set of ingredients and alchemizing them into a budding fertilized egg, zygote, eventually an embryo, and eventually a

---

* Find Paige Hasballah on social media @deltavenus.

new human. Your sacral energy point that holds your sexuality and your uterus also holds your creative fire.

There is an ironic and nonsensical tendency in westernized culture to look at pregnant folks as fragile, untouchable, virginal. The problematic, patriarchal roots of this is a whole other book in and of itself, but it's worth making note of so you can intentionally reject it, if you so choose. Pregnancy itself can ignite an increase in sexual interest. This of course won't be the case for everyone, as some folks experience the exact opposite for various reasons.

Being in touch with what sexuality looks like for you—in whatever way makes you feel most free—will be your ally in pregnancy, particularly when it comes time to open and release your sacral energy point to birth your baby through that particular portal. Instilling fear and uncertainty about tapping into our sexuality during pregnancy and birth has worked as a puritanical, patriarchal tool to strip birthing folks of a significant source of their power and autonomy during conception, pregnancy, and birth. Thus, in turn, this can require more reliance on the patriarchally rooted medical model to birth your baby.

The same hormones (prostaglandins) that are used in a medical induction are also found in semen. The same uterine contractions that your body will utilize during labor are available in every orgasm. Oxytocin—the hormone that dictates when your labor will begin, helps keep labor progressing, and naturally mitigates the perception of pain in labor—also just so happens to be the hormone that your body releases in high amounts during sex and orgasm. The delicate state of brainwaves that are your ally in birth, that get you to a meditative state where pain might not be perceived as "pain" at all, are also the same brainwaves you regularly tap into during sex with yourself or with a partner. And that's just naming a few ways our sexuality is our ally during birth—there are so many more.

A relationship with your sexuality is neither accessible nor desirable to everyone, so I'm by no means saying that a connection with your sexuality is going to make or break your birth experience. But the Ace of Wands (and many of the wands in general) is asking us to not let puritanical social conditioning be the reason why we aren't utilizing our sexuality to our advantage during conception, pregnancy, and birth.

⊰ ACE OF WANDS THEMES ⊱

beginnings, the element of fire, sacral chakra, creative spark, being ignited, embarking on a sexual journey, new ideas, what lights you up

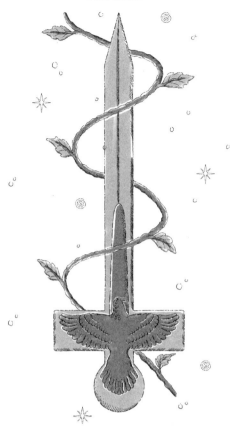

ACE OF SWORDS

You are being given the gift of a mental journey, which means you can trust yourself to make decisions from a logical place, and you can also expect the health of your brain chemistry to be tested for the sake of you learning more about how your brain works.

Naturally, when we're working with intellect, we're talking about brain chemistry, and when we're talking about brain chemistry, we are acknowledging all the ways that could go—fear, depression, clarity, indecisiveness, hesitancy, or coldness.

It's easy in the Ace of Swords to loosen our grip on our inner voice, because we think we're doing everything "by the book," so why check in with our intuition? This particular Ace needs the balance of the emotion-based thinking we receive from the cups and the root-based thinking offered by the pentacles, otherwise it can be too logical for its own good.

To put it simply, if you're making decisions about your pregnancy and birth based solely on numbers, statistics, and what society thinks, but you're smothering your own inner voice in order to justify that and make sense of the logic, then those choices are anything but logical because they're one-sided.

One major way the imbalanced manifestation of the Ace of Swords shows up is in how obsessively we consider and integrate recommendations or contraindications in what we should or shouldn't be taking into our bodies when we're pregnant. The studies are ever-changing and often not the whole picture. Often, they're recommendations not tailored to our specific bodies, because it's unethical to do double-blind studies on pregnant people. Herbalism is a highly useful resource for pregnancy nutrition that goes largely untapped because the FDA won't test and approve most herbs. For this reason, if you're researching herbs on Google, you won't be getting the whole picture, so curiosity and intuition are the appropriate balance to this truth-seeking, clear-cut energy. Inversely, there are several herbs commonly used in pregnancy that are doled out as good-for-everyone treatment, when no one thing is ever necessarily good or okay for everyone. No matter what, an individualized look at health and nutrition is necessary.

As you might guess, this card is an excellent tool when beginning to embark on the journey of educating yourself about your pregnancy and birth and will be a useful tool in making the decisions that will craft your birth plan. Again, just be careful that all that evidence-based education isn't smothering an intuitive knowing your body is trying to communicate with you.

While the energy of the Ace of Swords can be an ally and a protective measure, remember that it's also a weapon to be wielded with care. This card represents truth, but one can find almost any statistic to support the "truth" of anything that you might choose to believe. This energy has the dangerous potential of being a tool of manipulation or protecting the status quo, especially when not rooted in a relationship with intuition or a deep accountability practice.

Pay attention to where this card shows up in your spread (if you're doing a spread). Where is the sword pointing? In its imagery, is the tip of the sword exposed and ready to cut, or disarmed/sheathed? Is this card showing up representing a way that you are acting/thinking, or is it how someone else is trying to persuade you? Interrogating these kinds of questions will all be helpful in ensuring that your sword is being wielded with compassionate clarity, rather than rigid close-mindedness or manipulation.

⊰ ACE OF SWORDS THEMES ⊱

beginnings, the element of air, throat and third eye chakras, embarking on a journey
of intellectual expansion, brain chemistry, fears and anxieties,
how we communicate, sharp clarity, truth

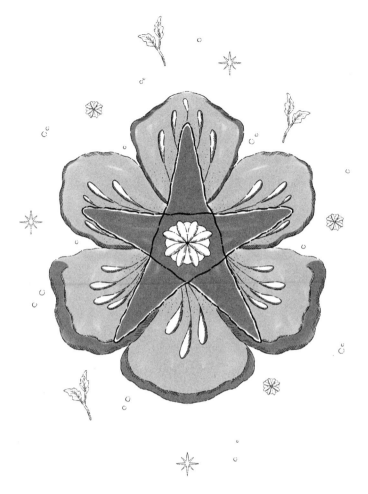

ACE OF PENTACLES

You are being given a seed, and what that will blossom and sprout into one day is yet to be determined. So, your only work in this Ace is to plant the seed.

Traditionally, many of the Aces can read as if something is happening *to* you, or something that you're receiving, instead of something that requires your active participation, but actually all the Aces require your receptivity, your grasping, your opening, and in the case of the Ace of Pentacles, your planting.

When you decided you were going to start trying to have a baby, you might've gotten off birth control and then thought that was that and started trying. What's the rush? Tend to your emotional and physical body first.* Feed yourself warm,

....

* I highly recommend the book *Awakening Fertility* by Heng Ou for more holistic information on the traditional path to preparing the body for pregnancy.

nutritious meals. Start building up your nutrient stores with nutritious herbs and whole foods *now* if you can, so that way when you are pregnant, your body has some nutrients to share with your baby.

Conscious preconception can be pivotal in how your pregnancy and birth go. By building up your nutritional stores so you don't get depleted, you can even help mitigate nausea once you do become pregnant. Pentacles deal with the earth, and therefore the physical body, reflecting plant vitamins and minerals that will nourish and sustain you and your baby throughout this process and well into parenthood.

If you've found yourself unexpectedly pregnant (for better or worse, for joy or terror), you might have been focused initially on the idea of a fully bloomed baby flower, wondering how that additional human would fit in to your already-full life, or if you even wanted to allow your body to be opened up for occupancy at all. Again, even in this scenario, we're jumping ahead. The Ace of Pentacles grounds you back down into the needs of your physical body right now.*

The Ace of Pentacles might be either confronting or comforting as you realize that the work of growing a human is *slow* work. At the very onset, you'll be about ten months from integrating that additional human into your life, if you agree to be occupied at all. And if you do agree to be occupied by that seed, letting it take up residence and nutrients from your cells, you still have to plant, water, and wait. The seed in the Ace of Pentacles isn't a big blooming flower yet, any more than an implanted mass of rapidly dividing cells isn't yet a baby. Patience, steady attention, watering, and nutrients are what are called for here, as well as deep noticing and honoring of what is happening for your mind and heart in all this.

Pentacles get their own special explanation for me. It's my favorite suit, and I think it requires more nuance than just being "of the earth." The first four points of a pentacle represent the four elements: water (cups, and therefore emotions), air (swords, and therefore mentality), fire (wands, and therefore creativity and sexuality), and earth (pentacles, the physical body). But the fifth point of the pentacle is you—the energy and magic of what it is to be human—your life force. You are so magically capable of connecting all those four elements and alchemizing them into something, even alchemizing those four elements into *a whole new human.*

Your sacral energy point that holds your creativity, sexuality, and womb is your

....

* Side note: both your heart and your brain are also parts of your physical body, and connecting with the needs of your emotional body, and mental health, are also going to be helpful in supporting your decision as to whether you want to move forward with sharing your body with another person or not, especially if your pregnancy discovery was unexpected.

fire. Your blood is your water. The oxygen you breathe that nourishes your cells is your air. The food you take in with all its nutrients and minerals is your earth. And you are freaking Elsa in *Frozen II*, the fifth magical element, taking all those ingredients and eventually making a baby out of them. Step into your power by rooting into this truth, and don't forget it.

ᦕ ACE OF PENTACLES THEMES ᦖ

beginnings, element of earth, root chakra, how all the elements are brought together, nutrition, planting the seed, tending to your body, building a human from scratch

NAUSEA TEA

"Herbs aren't designed to work as a remedy whilst you continue to violate the basic rules of your body. They act as a helping hand to give your body the support it needs to heal. They work best when you listen to your body and give it what it needs."

—Sophia Forrester, BSc MCPP, medical herbalist

Overall, I am of the belief that each symptom of pregnancy, whether perceived as positive or negative, is here to teach us something or is attempting to ask you for something, and therefore ought to be listened to and honored instead of swept away or brushed off as an inconvenience. So, this recipe for helping ease nausea will not necessarily make your nausea go away instantly and entirely or allow you to go on about your life as though you aren't a pregnant person. Plants are our allies, and they are too good of friends to let us miss out on the lesson that is nausea.

As such, when you brew yourself this tea, you're still going to need to do your part (as much as you are able to, and your life/job allows) and slow the fuck down. Nausea is aggravated by sudden movements and not honoring and prioritizing rest. Like I said, symptoms are often trying to communicate a need, and with nausea, it can be communicating a nutrient deficiency (which is where the following herbal infusion recipe can help). Nausea is aggravated by having meals far apart instead of small meals more frequently.

I know it's not accessible to every pregnant person to "slow down," but consider how ableist and capitalistically rooted is the perpetual, steady insistence on productivity. In any of the ways that you can reject that, I implore you to try. Pregnant people need to be able to take up space in more ways than just getting a priority seat on the train when they're thirty-eight weeks pregnant. It may be possible to start conditioning the people around us to honor the uncomfortable transitions we're going through and taking up space to rest.

Some of these ingredients directly reduce nausea, while others are nutrient-supportive, which will help quell the nausea by giving your body the nutrients it's asking for. That being said, if every ingredient is not readily accessible to you, work with what you have—something is better than nothing.

While drinking your tea, eat a protein-rich snack like nuts, oatmeal, or bone broth, stay hydrated, and try to rest. Nausea really sucks, I know. I'm not trying to bypass that truth or romanticize something that, for a while, can be really disruptive to our lives.

Nausea is a common symptom during labor. Your body knows this, and it's trying to prepare you for this kind of discomfort. This human you're working on growing *will* disrupt your life in every way possible and, postpartum, will pin you to your couch for different reasons. Transitions are uncomfortable, babies are disruptive—with this unwelcome symptom, even this early on, your body is preparing you.

Now finally, here to accompany and bolster the effects of rest on relieving nausea, a recipe:

INGREDIENTS

*1 Tbsp dried red raspberry leaf**

2 tsp dried nettles

1 tsp ginger (fresh or dried)

1 tsp mint (fresh or dried, but add a little more if you're using fresh)

1 tsp dried chamomile

1 tsp dried lemon balm

Fresh lemon juice and honey (optional)

DIRECTIONS

Add the red raspberry leaf, nettles, ginger, mint, chamomile, and lemon balm to a tea strainer and steep in hot water for 5 minutes (any longer won't hurt, but it may develop a bitter taste). Adding your desired amount of fresh lemon and honey to taste will help with any aversions to the tea that you might be feeling as a result of your nausea. I also find drinking my tea iced helps it go down easier if I'm already feeling nauseated.

---

* Note: If you have endometriosis, polycystic ovary syndrome (PCOS), or uterine fibroids, do not use red raspberry leaf, or products like this that contain red raspberry leaf, as the estrogen present in it could worsen the symptoms of those conditions.

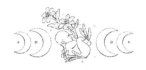

THE TWOS

❧ MONTH 2 THEMES ❧

cell division, becoming more than one, putting into action the gift presented in the Aces, partnerships, making decisions, weighing two sides, the discomfort of transformation

IN THE PHYSICAL BODY

Your embryo is the size of a pea in month 2 and rapidly developing all those things your pregnancy app or book is telling you about (some internal organs, muscles, hair, fingernails, etc.). That means *you*—your body is alchemizing all these brand-new body parts for this embryo. *Wild*, right?

Ever since I was a pregnant person myself, I've found it ironic that we culturally tend to make accommodations for pregnant folks who are very visibly pregnant, but some of the toughest work is in this beginning part, the part that no one can see, and often before we've even told people we're pregnant.

It's not unusual in the first trimester to have a racing heart or feel a shortness of breath as if you've been doing cardio when you haven't—this is because your body is working in overdrive to lay the foundational building blocks of what will become your baby's body. Also, progesterone is still playing a star role at this point, and progesterone is a sedative, so this can also account for sleepiness or sluggishness.

If you haven't visited it already, see the nausea tea recipe (page 39) to learn about why slowing down and honoring this transition is what's called for right now. This will likely be the first of many ways your coming child will disrupt your life and teach you how to truly rest.

TWO OF CUPS

Whether you do or don't have a romantic partner in pregnancy, you do have a partner, and that partner is the embryo you're growing. You're never in this alone; you're doing this thing entirely together in an unseen dance. People can feel your belly (if you choose to let them) but only *you* are on this forty-plus-week-long date with your baby, having the opportunity to get to know them inside and out.

Try to think about how they're experiencing this whole gestation thing. If you experience a stress response, or a sudden burst of adrenaline or cortisol, they experience it too. So do something to counteract it. Speak to them and tell them they're not actually in danger (to them, they don't know the difference between adrenaline caused by mortal danger or if it's just because you got called into your boss's office or you watched a scary movie). If you can, do something that creates the hormones that will balance out intensity, such as laughing, positive touching, eating your favorite foods, or taking a nap. Be considerate of what your little partner is feeling throughout pregnancy. This is the medicine of the Two of Cups—to recognize pregnancy for the partnership that it is.

In the Two of Cups, we are taught that we learn the most about ourselves through our relationships with others, how we reflect off them, both our differences and similarities. We define ourselves through how we brush up against, push, and pull against one another in relationship. So, this card is an invitation to look for that—in all relationships with your partner, your friends, and now, with your children, expected and current. Children have a beautiful and maddening tendency to shed light on what we like to cover up, such as repressed trauma, and yes, it starts even this early in utero.

I call it beautiful because they are casting light on what needs to be seen so it can be healed, but that is not to trivialize this work. It is deep and difficult and should be undergone with care and probably appropriate guidance from a mental health professional depending on your situation. If you are someone who experienced trauma or abuse in your childhood, your very own children will trigger you, because you will see your own small, innocent self in them. This is the exact reflection I'm talking about with the Two of Cups. It is an opportunity to heal.

❧ TWO OF CUPS THEMES ❧
healing, being in partnership with your baby, related to the Lovers card, using your relationships with others as a mirror for yourself, growth and self-understanding through relating to others

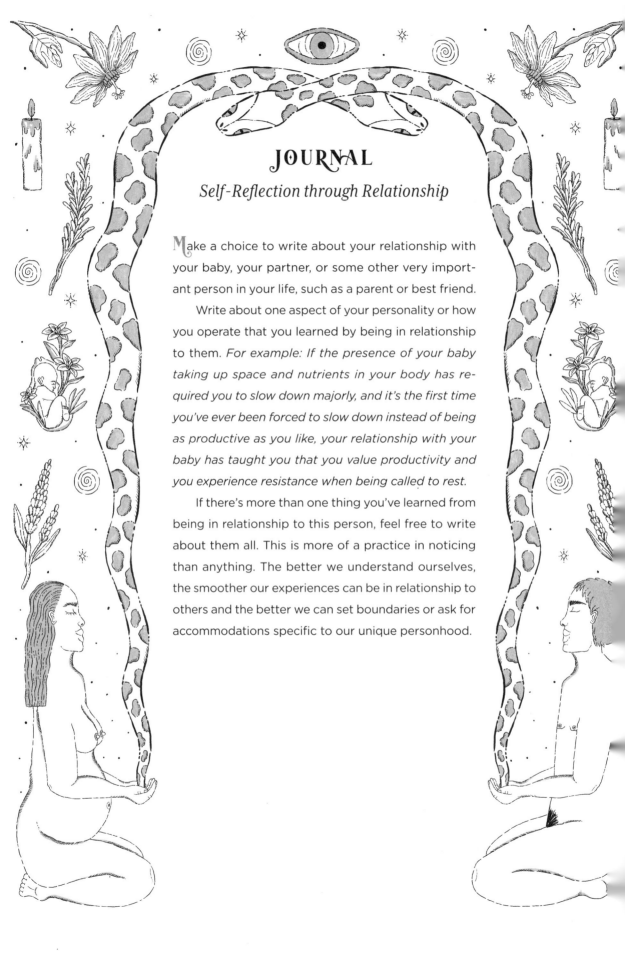

JOURNAL

Self-Reflection through Relationship

Make a choice to write about your relationship with your baby, your partner, or some other very important person in your life, such as a parent or best friend.

Write about one aspect of your personality or how you operate that you learned by being in relationship to them. *For example: If the presence of your baby taking up space and nutrients in your body has required you to slow down majorly, and it's the first time you've ever been forced to slow down instead of being as productive as you like, your relationship with your baby has taught you that you value productivity and you experience resistance when being called to rest.*

If there's more than one thing you've learned from being in relationship to this person, feel free to write about them all. This is more of a practice in noticing than anything. The better we understand ourselves, the smoother our experiences can be in relationship to others and the better we can set boundaries or ask for accommodations specific to our unique personhood.

TWO OF WANDS

The spark of the creative journey you were gifted in the Ace of Wands needs some plans, don't you think? Anxiety over what the parenthood path means for you with this pregnancy can be satisfied by making plans and putting them into action.

By now you are likely meeting with and interviewing health care providers. Check in and make sure that you feel balanced, centered, and calm in your body when you're around them. When you're interviewing potential midwives or OBs, check in with your body. Do you feel tension anywhere? Does your throat feel open and comfortable to speak freely, or does it close up and feel unsafe to ask questions? Are your hands clenched around them or open and relaxed? Are you slumping in posture to protect your heart, or are you confident in taking up time and space in their office with trust that they are happy to spend this time on you? What does eye contact with them feel like?

Making and implementing plans can be overwhelming and daunting, especially if you are now feeling those early pregnancy symptoms. Two of Wands energy is great for asking for help if you need it to start working on those plans. Allow what you're not good at to be balanced out by what someone else is naturally good at, whether that be your partner, a close friend, or a trusted family member.

⸙ TWO OF WANDS THEMES ⸙

acting upon your ideas, setting plans in motion, having choices, self-trust

TAROT SPREAD FOR CHOOSING A HEALTH CARE PROVIDER

What message, if any, am I not paying attention to when I am with this potential care provider?

What message is my body telling me when I am with this potential care provider?

What will I learn/can I expect from continuing to work with this care provider?

Is this care provider the best choice available to me right now?

Pull a card for a message from your guides regarding your current care provider.

TWO OF SWORDS

The Two of Swords can look like doubling down because we thought we knew everything there was to know about some pregnancy-related thing, and we are being confronted with the fact that maybe we did not.

Watching popular TV shows and movies that have birth scenes is not childbirth education. In fact, unfortunately, I have yet to ever see a cinematic rendition of a birth scene that was remotely accurate to what real birth is, whether medicalized or physiologic birth. And that's a shame, because media input does have real impacts on our perceptions and expectations, impacts that calcify into beliefs that can be very deeply rooted and hard to recognize and extract. Yet for many of us, popular media will be the only visual representations of birth that we will ever be introduced to.

In the Two of Swords, our ego doesn't want to admit that we don't know things, so we choose to stay willfully ignorant, despite knowing that we have more to learn. This is understandable, and it's simply your brain trying to keep you safe—if you don't know everything about pregnancy and birth, then that means you signed up for one big unknown experience, and especially for folks who've experienced trauma, there is nothing romantic or cute about the idea of a "big unknown." But even though it's understandable, it doesn't mean we need to be ruled by the fear-based desire to know everything already.

Remember the curiosity suggested by the Ace of Swords. Call it in and let it humble you. It's easy to become frozen in this energy because it has an air of stubbornness to it. There's no shame in learning more and then integrating what you've learned into how you'll move forward.

Seek out podcasts that share all kinds of birth stories, and not just traumatic emergency events.* Watch birth videos online of normal physiologic birth to get a feel for what it's really like. And then start keeping your eye out for childbirth education classes in the future (preferably a class that isn't affiliated with your birthing place, so you aren't subject to bias in their teachings).

☽ TWO OF SWORDS THEMES ☾

stubbornness, our perceptions of the truth being skewed by what we hold to be true, difficult decision-making, boundaries, more knowledge and planning as an antidote to anxiety

TWO OF PENTACLES

The realization that you're pregnant can put you on pause for a moment. When you start rerouting your nutrition and self-care to be more conscious of the additional human you have on board, it can feel as if Pregnant Person is your only job title now in the Ace of Pentacles.

But in the Two of Pentacles, you get to figure out how to be both a pregnant person *and* whatever other roles you play. This Two is a call to juggle both and also to recognize how good of a job you're doing being a pregnant person and wearing all your other hats, especially if you are already parenting other children.

We have such unrealistic expectations of pregnant people that when we ourselves are pregnant, experiencing shortness of breath, nausea, fatigue, backaches, and all the other possible ailments so much earlier than we expected, we think that we should be able to do more at this stage, simply because our body might not yet have gone through the visible, physical change of acquiring a pregnant-looking belly.

But I'm here to tell you that, given the circumstances, you're juggling your life

------

* The podcast *Birthful* by Adriana Lozada is a wonderful resource both for birth stories and evidence-based, balanced information about pregnancy and birth.

and being a pregnant person beautifully—even if that juggling looks like setting new boundaries with work or other commitments, paring down, or maybe keeping all your pre-pregnancy commitments afloat just fine. The point is, just know that whatever you're doing, and how much you're doing of it, is more than enough.

☽ TWO OF PENTACLES THEMES ☾

only juggling what you physically can, paring down, the physical body being less capable than usual, always growing even when it looks like you're "doing nothing"

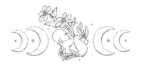

THE THREES

MONTH 3 (WEEKS 9 TO 13)

"Surround yourself with people who trust your strengths and see the warrior in your vulnerability."
—Erika M. Pérez Latorre, holistic birth companion*

⊰ MONTH 3 THEMES ⊱
building community, self-discovery and self-love, sitting with intense and difficult emotions, sitting with uncomfortable physical symptoms and learning from them, putting in the work

IN THE PHYSICAL BODY

In the beginning of the third month, your "wombmate" is an embryo, and later in this same month they'll start to be considered a fetus. Your embryo is about the size of a lime now, and even more active (though it's rare that you will feel their movements at this point, it's totally possible).

At the start of this month, you'll likely still be very much in the nausea and fatigue stage (if those are symptoms you've been experiencing), but there are better days ahead (fingers crossed!). Toward the end of your third month, when you shift into the second trimester, some of that hormonal overdrive that your body was

....

* Find Erika at birthingundisturbed.com and on social media @birthingundisturbed.

producing to hang on to your embryo hopefully won't need to be in high gear anymore, and it will start to level out.

THREE OF CUPS

This card shows up as a call for you to start finding your community, or if you're lucky enough to have found one, this is a nudge to lean on it. Community is everything in the work of bringing new humans into the world, and you won't be doing anyone any favors in trying to isolate yourself or thinking that you're strong enough to go it alone.

Of course, it's not always our own personal choice whether we are in it alone or not, but it's time to start thinking about finding and building a relationship with a community sturdy enough to lean on, if you don't feel like you have that already. Nurture them mutually as much as you can and allow yourself to feel comfortable to be nourished by them too.

Colonialism thrives off and perpetuates individualistic culture* and will try to cast shame on the ideas of collective care or anything other than the nuclear family model that colonial white-supremacist capitalism favors. So, when you feel shame coming up, trying to keep you from reaching out and keeping you isolated, know that it is a revolutionary act to push through that shame and declare your human right to your community. It is particularly revolutionary for Black pregnant folks, Indigenous pregnant folks, and every other culture that has been historically and currently underserved by colonial ideals to reach out and reclaim this right to community.

If you find yourself feeling uncomfortable with that kind of asking or receiving—don't just leave it at discomfort, explore why. This is important work; it could be a whole book in and of itself, and it's one I'm not qualified to write† being that my ancestry is the primary beneficiary of colonialism's oppressive legacy. But staying curious and exploring enough to find community is huge, important work that

....

* A concept I've learned repeatedly in different iterations from different antiracism or decolonial teachers such as Layla F. Saad and Dr. Rosales Meza. Individualism feeds into capitalism, because when folks don't have community to lean on, they must buy more things out of convenience, but an individualistic life without help and community care isn't tenable for longterm living and thriving.

† But I do recommend the book *We Live for the We* by Dani McClain on the topic of Black motherhood and what that historically and culturally means and has represented for the community.

doesn't benefit you alone—it's shifting an oppressive paradigm for the legacy you're carrying out as well.

꒰ **THREE OF CUPS THEMES** ꒱

*soul friends, calling in community, receiving support, emotional growth,
building your village*

EXERCISE

BRAINSTORMING FOR VILLAGE BUILDING

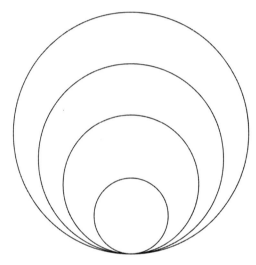

In the smallest circle draw you and your baby (or write your names).

The circle that surrounds you and your baby is your "inner circle." Here, write the names of any adult who lives in your house who is capable of giving support (partners, parents, siblings, roommates, aunts, etc.).

The third circle represents your greater community. Add the names of close friends and family members who don't live with you but are willing to support you in your pregnancy journey and postpartum.

The outermost circle represents your external support. Write in the names of all your hired professionals—midwife, doctor, doula, therapist, chiropractor, acupuncturist, pelvic floor therapist, massage therapist, tarot reader.

Once you've completed the exercise and written down all the names, don't judge what's there, just notice.

You'll likely see that the number of names grows as your circles go outward. If not, start thinking of what conversations need to happen with your inner circle and your greater community so that they know your needs and expectations for how they show up for you on this journey in pregnancy and postpartum.

If the outer circle representing your external support is looking scant, let's make a plan. Can you ask someone from the other two circles to help support funding one of these services? How can we integrate an option in your baby registry to fund these kinds of external support systems? Can you reach out to certain practitioners to see if they offer sliding-scale services or accept insurance? Don't let that outer ring of support go unoccupied for fear of asking.

THREE OF WANDS

You're outgrowing something, and it's not just your prepregnancy clothing. It's time to pare down and streamline, so get curious about what that would look like.

This will be different for everyone, so I'll provide some examples: If you're a business owner, but you're all over the place, pare down your offerings and keep only what lights you up and keeps you and your family financially safe—you don't need it all, you just need enough when it comes to bringing humans into the world. If you're in a friendship that is energetically laborious to maintain, and they aren't honoring where you are in this pregnancy, in this life, it might be time to limit the amount of time and energy you give to that friendship, perhaps cutting them out completely if that is what's called for. Those are just a couple examples of the paring down that the Three of Wands might be asking for.

Basically, whatever integrity-based and minimalist decisions you make right now will be the right decisions. You don't need to be aggressive or contemptuous about this paring down, because ultimately what you're releasing likely helped you see a new perspective (even if that new perspective was only learning how to cut people/things out of your life—that's a valuable lesson too!).

This is also a point in your pregnancy where, if you are choosing a medicalized birth route, you might be offered many different tests at varying degrees of necessity. This is an appropriate moment to tap into and listen to what your intuition has to say. Research the accuracy of evidence-based information or each test offered to you before you consent. In medicalized birth, the care is standardized, not necessarily based on individual risk level or environmental factors, and though no one might ever tell you this throughout pregnancy, these tests are actually optional—all of them.

In this case, when your level of stress matters so much, less is more. Sometimes test results (whether they're accurate or not) can have the potential to change the trajectory of the kind of care you receive and the kind of birth decisions your care provider recommends, not to mention the severe toll it can take on your mental health throughout the rest of your pregnancy. This is an incredibly important time to pick up that thread of intuitive knowledge and make your decisions from that intuitive place that only you know for your body and your fetus. You are a client, not a patient—take up space and feel empowered to customize your care based on what you actually want and need, knowing that you always have options.

ᛉ THREE OF WANDS THEMES ᛊ

outgrowing old ways of being, paring down who you allow in your inner circle, simplifying, planning, making decisions from a place of integrity

THREE OF SWORDS

By the end of the third month of pregnancy, you'll be transitioning out of your first trimester, into your second trimester. If life hasn't taught you this already, pregnancy, birth, postpartum, and parenting will surely teach you that transitions are hard. This card is the most emotional/watery card in the very mental suit of swords. The feelings are likely heavy, intense, and somber, even painful.

Whatever is causing your specific difficulty right now is less important than just allowing yourself to fully feel it, without shying away. Big important disclaimer: I do not associate any card in the tarot with actual miscarriage or infant loss, not even the Death card, and therefore I am *not* saying this card is indicative of miscarriage. *Please note this!*

As someone who has experienced miscarriage, I know I would be remiss not to honor this heartbreaking experience. The painful feelings of loss and betrayal that this card represents are the feelings that one likely experiences if loss has ever wedged its way into your story. If you experience loss of any kind, whether that manifests as your favorite care provider not being available anymore, a miscarriage, an abortion, a friendship revealing its true and unsupportive nature during your pregnancy, the loss of a loved one, or maybe learning of a condition that shoots your dreams of a home birth—whatever the case may be, this card tells us to be real with what that grief is, recognize it as grief, give it all the space and tears, and talk and move through and with it as often as that grief needs your attention.

In my deepest, darkest Three of Swords moment I've ever experienced in my life, this wisdom came to me: *When people say they feel dead inside, I think they actually mean that they feel* too alive *for comfort.* I'm not romanticizing pain or any other difficult emotions; this is simply a neutral reality—that pain reminds us of our mortality, our aliveness. This is why we pinch ourselves when something feels unreal.

Without bypassing the pain, I hope I can share with you the healing balm that this card can be. There will be an eventual shift out of this intensity of feeling. And in that way, this card is a beautiful teacher to prepare us for labor and birth. We don't get over pain, we move through and with it. We don't let go of perceived "negative" emotions, we integrate them, and eventually allow them to live alongside our joy, peace, excitement, and hope for the future.

❧ THREE OF SWORDS THEMES ☙

being let down, heartaches resurfacing, transition into second trimester, emotional intensity, loss in some form, learning the purpose of pain

THREE OF PENTACLES

This seed has been planted for nine to twelve weeks now, and it's still only this tiny sprout?! I know. It feels unfair, and the "over it" feeling can be compounded by the fact that you might still be very much in the worst of your first-trimester pregnancy symptoms.

This phase, too, is a part of the slow but steady work of human building. This is work you can't rush. There are lessons in slowing down, lessons in listening to your body, and lessons in what nutrients your body is asking for to be found in all those yucky first-trimester symptoms. As much as your life allows, do what your body asks.

Now is a good time to start building your birth team if you haven't already (if this card is coming up for you, it might indicate that you haven't built that team yet or that your team might need some restructuring). You might have your chosen midwife or OB squared away by now, but think about the rest of the birth team. Will you have a doula or a knowledgeable, helpful family member? Do you want a photographer? A supportive sibling? A grandparent in the background of your homebirth cooking you soup for postpartum? Keep the team small but mighty, streamlined, and useful. Make sure everyone that's going to be there is intending to show up in a *helpful* capacity, not just to observe their new family member enter the world. Make sure that everyone that's going to be there is going to bring a calm and trusting energy of the safety and normalness to the birth, not bringing erratic, fearful energy into your birth space.

Birth is not for everybody and their mother, birth is for *you*—what support *you* need, what *you* would feel comforted by, who *you* would feel comfortable being vulnerable around. (Hint: These are good rules to live by when choosing who will come to help you postpartum as well—not to visit, but to help and support you.)

⊰ THREE OF PENTACLES THEMES ⊱

seeds planted starting to be visible sprouts, the slow work of building something from scratch, building your team, collaboration

NOURISHING
PREGNANCY INFUSION

Infusions are a great, highly absorbable, and bioavailable way for your body to receive the nutrients it needs to assist your body in the work of human building. *Note: Herbs are rarely, if ever, evaluated by the FDA, meaning that many things not proven to be safe are just that—not proven, because they have not been tested by medicalized standards. Without offering you medical advice, herbal knowledge is something all our ancestors had and knew how to wield effectively to meet certain bodily needs. Whenever I'm suggesting recipes in this book, it's in a generalized manner. In order to say for sure whether or not an herbal recipe is safe for you specifically, I (or preferably a certified herbalist or naturopathic doctor) would need to talk to you about your specific body and its needs. Consult a trained herbalist or naturopathic doctor if you're not sure and do your own research knowing your own body and/or your particular drug contraindications, or if you trust them, consult your care provider, stay updated on new information when it is found, and make an informed decision for yourself from there.*

Red raspberry leaf is probably the most common herb you've heard of for pregnancy—this plant friend offers B vitamins, vitamin C, antioxidants, potassium, magnesium, zinc, phosphorus, and iron (though it should be noted that this herb may be contraindicated if you have polycystic ovary syndrome, fibroids, or endometriosis).* Alfalfa is the red raspberry leaf's balanced counterpart with vitamins A, D, E, and K (the vitamin K makes its medicine really shine later in pregnancy because it may help prevent postpartum hemorrhage). Nettles are high in vitamins A, C, and K and also have potassium, iron, and calcium. Oatstraw is rich in calcium, B vitamins, manganese, and zinc. All these minerals and nutrients contribute to a multitude of things from easing nausea, to toning the uterus in preparation for labor, to building your blood's iron levels, to easing anxiety and tension, and more.

INGREDIENTS

1 Tbsp red raspberry leaf

1 Tbsp alfalfa

1 Tbsp nettles

1 Tbsp oatstraw

(or a handful of premade mixture of the above herbs)

Blackstrap molasses for sweetening (optional)

Lemonade for serving (optional)

DIRECTIONS

Heat a couple of quarts of water in a glass or stainless-steel pot over high heat, and once it comes to a boil, turn off the heat, add your herbs, stir, and then cover with a lid. I use about a tablespoon of each, or if I've mixed all these herbs together ahead of time, I'll use a big handful of the herb mixture.

. . . .

* Red raspberry leaf is so popular that it's often recommended without looking at a person's individual health, and it is thanks to Mayte Noguez, a traditional *sobadora*, that I now know that there are times when red raspberry leaf might not be recommended for everyone. For more informative content like that about womb health, you can support her on Patreon and follow her on Instagram @maytethewombdoula.

Allow the herbs to steep in the hot water until the water isn't super-hot anymore, for at least 2 hours but up to 12. This is an infusion, not a tea, so the long steeping time is with the intention of extracting the maximum amount of nutritional benefits out of the herbs.

Using a cheesecloth or clean, thin towel, strain the liquid into the glass container of your choice. Squeeze the cloth to get every last drop of nutrients out of those plant friends.

You can sweeten this infusion with blackstrap molasses for an added iron boost. This infusion is medicine though, so it can be bitter. Because of this, I always cut my infusions with lemonade (I know this isn't a nutritiously perfect solution, but it got me to drink the healthy stuff, so I offered myself grace in that department—you do you). This should last in the refrigerator for up to a week.

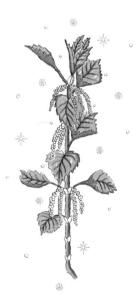

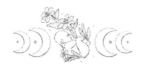

THE FOURS

❧ MONTH 4 THEMES ❧

emerging from the first trimester feeling better and more balanced, a period of respite after the discomforts of the previous months, look up, look around, and feel gratitude for the gift of feeling good again, expansion, consistency

IN THE PHYSICAL BODY

It's common to feel your fetus's movements for the first time in this time period. This can feed into the "snapping out of it" energy of the Fours, reminding and giving us renewed purpose for all the symptoms we just endured during the first trimester without a tangible return on investment just yet.

Nervous system functions are developing more now, which means your baby is likely starting to hear better and sensing the vibrations of your voice. You might be someone whose body is visibly "showing" at this point, and you might not be. Despite what the media and modern medicine caters to, pregnancy doesn't look only one way, and however you feel in relation to your body right now is totally valid and worthy of giving space to.

If it hasn't started already, round ligament* and/or lower back pain might ramp up as the hormone relaxin is produced, relaxing the muscle that holds your uterus in place to make room and to allow your pelvis more flexibility as it prepares your body for birth.

....

* The round ligament supports the uterus, and round ligament pain is felt along the lower front of the abdomen. This pain can be felt on both sides or just one side.

Back pain and round ligament pain isn't something you just need to grin, bear, and endure all throughout your pregnancy. If chiropractic care is accessible to you, seeking it out or continuing that relationship will be highly beneficial to the way your body feels now and throughout your entire pregnancy and can help prepare your body for labor. Look for a chiropractor who specializes in the Webster technique, which is the special method of adjustments that should be used on pregnant people to prepare their bodies for birth and bodyfeeding.

If a chiropractor is not accessible to you, there are bodily movements and exercises* to incorporate into your daily life that can mimic the comforting benefits of a chiropractic adjustment:

- Cat/cow: On your hands and knees, tilt your pelvis under while you tuck your chin (cat), then rotate your pelvis up while you lift your chin (cow); do thirty reps before bed every night, and as needed throughout the day for alleviating pressure on the lower back.

- Forward lunges (do before squats): Using the support of a sturdy piece of furniture, plant one foot forward and one foot back, and then bend at the knees to lunge forward. The point of these lunges isn't the balance, but deepening the stretch in the muscles at the front of your belly.

- Low squats: Place your feet a little wider than hip-width apart and lower into a deep squat (sometimes it's helpful to hold someone's hands, or hold on to a sturdy piece of furniture for support). Hold for as long as is comfortable. Sitting, bouncing, or circling your hips on a birth ball also works great if getting into a low squat is not accessible to you.

- Psoas release: Lying flat on your back, positioned near the edge of an elevated surface (such as a couch or a bed), allow one leg to relax back over the edge of the surface you're on, then pull a knee up alongside your belly and hold it there for a few breaths; repeat on the other side.

- Figure eights: These are great for when you're taking breaks on long car rides; stand up with your feet stably rooted, hands on your hips, and move your hips in a figure-eight motion.

- Forward-leaning inversion: To alleviate pressure on your lower back

* Some of these movements along with photo illustrations of how to do them can be found on the Spinning Babies website (www.spinningbabies.com), dedicated to helping people with optimal fetal position for labor.

and promote optimal positioning for the baby (more commonly used in the third trimester), clasp your hands and brace your elbows on the ground in front of you, then elevate your knees onto a higher surface behind you (such as a low couch) and hold for a few breaths or as long as is comfortable for your arms.

FOUR OF CUPS

You might be reveling in the sense of balanced serenity as a result of leaving some nasty symptoms behind in the first trimester. Or, if you're not leaving them behind yet, the Four of Cups asks us to not adopt a "woe is me" mindset here. As cliché and annoying as it may feel, there's a lot to be grateful for right now, but it can be hard to look around to notice it. Are things really as shitty as you think they are? Or have you been *in* that narrative for so long that you're committed to it, and can't see the forest for the trees? This card (and the tarot in general) doesn't cater to us when we're intentionally inhabiting our lower selves, so this card can feel like an unwelcome callout to some.

The energy of the Four of Cups is unsatisfied with everything and isn't noticing the abundance of blessings surrounding them as a result. If you find yourself inhabiting this stagnant energy, a good exercise is to literally, wherever you are, look up. Look up from this book. Look away from your phone, away from the TV, away from the project you're working on, away from whatever is immediately in front of you, and very slowly, mindfully, and thoroughly, take in what surrounds you. Maybe you're looking at food to eat, the walls of your home, your growing belly; maybe you're outside and looking at the miracle that is any single leaf, bug, flower, or animal.

If you pulled this card in a spread, pay attention to its position in the spread. Traditionally,* this card is represented by a person so focused on their three cups that they are looking forward and not noticing that a fourth cup is being divinely offered to them. If you are doing a spread, where else in your spread does that divine

....

* Note that whenever I say "traditionally" in reference to the imagery of a card, I'm likely referring to the depictions that Pamela Colman Smith illustrated for the Rider-Waite-Smith deck first created in 1909. This deck has become the standard upon which many (but not all) artists base their card depictions in modern tarot decks. You'll typically hear this deck referred to as the "Rider-Waite" tarot, as Arthur Waite supervised the deck's creation and wrote the guidebook, and William Rider & Son was the publisher. Pamela Colman Smith's name was not typically included in the title until relatively recently because she was a woman and because she was (purported to be) biracial, which, at the time of its publishing, made her pivotal involvement in the deck's creation largely unspoken.

cup look like it's "coming from"? What card is next to or above it in the spread? What other card in the spread is the figure focusing on?

Look, if those three cups you're already holding are really enough, no rush. There's no need to reach for a fourth cup (a new opportunity, a new solution, etc.), if you have your hands full with three. What is meant for you won't miss you.

❧ FOUR OF CUPS THEMES ❧

knowing when you already have enough on your plate, pausing, resting, waiting, gratitude for how far you've come

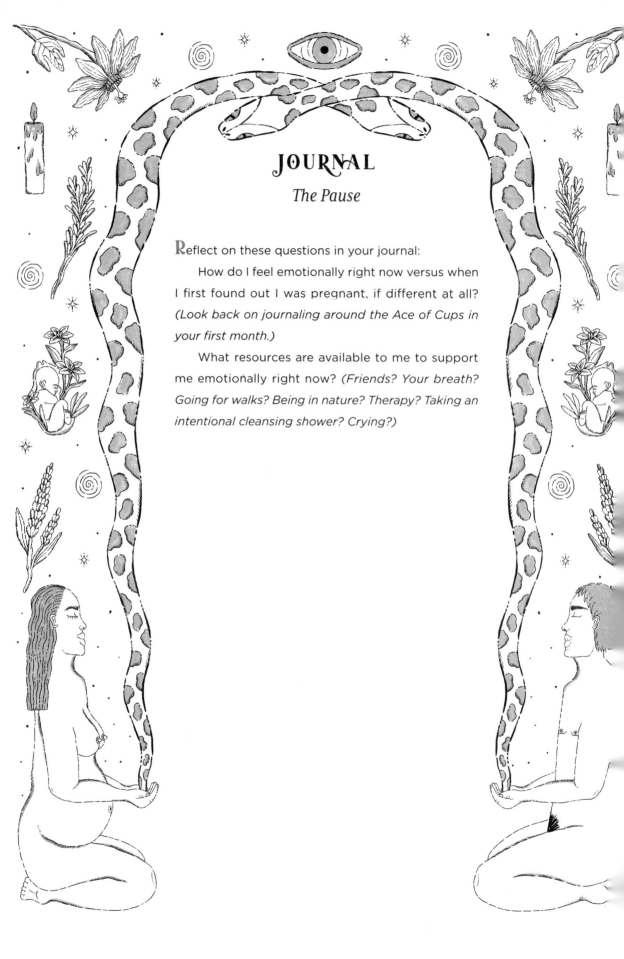

JOURNAL

The Pause

Reflect on these questions in your journal:

How do I feel emotionally right now versus when I first found out I was pregnant, if different at all? *(Look back on journaling around the Ace of Cups in your first month.)*

What resources are available to me to support me emotionally right now? *(Friends? Your breath? Going for walks? Being in nature? Therapy? Taking an intentional cleansing shower? Crying?)*

FOUR OF WANDS

If you're feeling good, and things are all feeling right, balanced, and in order, great! Let good be good. The energy of this card is sturdy and balanced, and there's a lot of journey left ahead, so pause and be grateful for a period of ease.

A great way to play into this card's energy, and exercise the creativity available in the wands, is to plan a gathering or a celebration. Not a baby shower, just a *Chocolat*-style dinner party with nourishing food and good company (if you don't know the movie reference, then just know that I am referring to an intimate gathering that nourishes both the body and soul). Invite the folks you adore who know you're pregnant and allow their excitement for your pregnancy to fill you up. It doesn't have to be an expensive or extravagant party, but just an intentional gathering to set the joyful tone for the people in your life so they can know what energy you're cultivating and expecting during this phase of your journey.

You did a lot of work to get to this point in pregnancy! I know that since your body does the work for you, it might not feel like "work," but remember that fatigue from the first trimester? (I mean, I hope it's a memory by now.) That was because of all the tangible, hard work your body was putting in to build a human from scratch. Honor the work that has been put in already to get you to this point and allow joy a seat at your table.

This card is an intentional respite along the way, celebrating how far you've come and acknowledging how much more road there is to travel.

⤫ FOUR OF WANDS THEMES ⤬
pausing to honor and celebrate, milestones, rest and respite on the journey, kindred community, not being able to see the end yet but honoring how far you've come

FOUR OF SWORDS

The swords are inactive in the fourth card of this suit, indicating laying down arms, rest, and rejuvenation. Right now is a good time to not make anything harder than it needs to be. Fighting for what we deserve will come later in the journey, but right now we need rest after the big contraction of the Three of Swords. We need to integrate the lessons of the Three, and integration requires rest, dreaming, and blank space.

Just because the worst of your nausea and fatigue are (hopefully) behind you doesn't mean to barrel back into business as usual and work just as hard as you did before pregnancy. Those lessons you gleaned from the first trimester are still true, and you need to prioritize rest whenever you can. If there are added stressors in your life (via social media, friendship drama, work drama, etc.), you have permission to disengage from those cortisol[*] producers for a while and regenerate.

There will be some stressors you can't necessarily just disengage from, such as the chronic weathering from living in a racist, capitalist, ableist society, particularly if you are of an identity that has been historically, systemically, and relentlessly marginalized. This makes it all the more important to disengage from the stressors you can choose to leave behind. Pregnancy is the time to protect your peace and prioritize yourself. That is enough.

I focus so much on prioritizing rest but not because pregnant people are fragile and can't or shouldn't be doing things and moving their bodies. I absolutely think they should, and, in most cases, pregnant people are capable of almost everything they were pre-pregnancy! I prioritize rest because our capitalistically driven, ableist, fat-phobic society has no problem pushing continued productivity during pregnancy, expecting your body to "bounce back" after birth, or even simply upholding the expectation that you can and should be just as productive and present at your job when your body is also working really hard in another way. These pressures are felt even more by BIPOC pregnant folks.[†] The space to choose rest and rejuvenation is not accessible to everyone, making choices to honor your body's need for rest even more revolutionary if and when you can make the space for it.

⊰ FOUR OF SWORDS THEMES ⊱

rest because the experience of the Three of Swords was heavy, rest for what's next in the Five, rough transitions ahead, realistic expectations for yourself, taking a break from what causes you stress

---

* According to the Mayo Clinic, "Cortisol, the primary stress hormone, increases sugars (glucose) in the bloodstream, enhances your brain's use of glucose and increases the availability of substances that repair tissues. Cortisol also curbs functions that would be nonessential or harmful in a fight-or-flight situation." ("Chronic Stress Puts Your Health at Risk," July 8, 2021, https://www.mayoclinic.org/healthy -lifestyle/stress-management/in-depth/stress/art-20046037).

† The Nap Ministry, with the motto "Rest is resistance," is a great, empowering, educational resource that focuses on the revolutionary importance of rest for Black Americans in particular. Find them online at www.thenapministry.wordpress.com and @thenapministry.

FOUR OF PENTACLES

This card is a call to make integrity-based decisions, in general, but particularly focused on financial decisions. Trust that there will be enough universal abundance for you when you make decisions from this place of integrity, even if you can't see it right now. Start imagining enough for yourself.

I know capitalism has yet to die, so lack of accessibility is not a figment of anyone's imagination, and not having enough is not because of a failure to manifest properly or think positively enough. But sometimes we've inhabited the idea of things not being accessible to us for so long that we don't look up and try to get creative about how we might be able to obtain the resources we need and deserve.

If you feel like you can't afford a doula because you're prioritizing expensive baby gadgets, it might be time to get real about what you're willing to give value to and why. If you truly can't afford a doula, have you assumed that's that and not considered doulas who offer sliding-scale or pro-bono services? If you're claiming you wish you could afford a midwife, but your insurance deductible is the same as (if not more than) the fee for the entirety of midwifery care, then examine the parts of you that hide behind frugality as an excuse to not think more critically about the possibilities. There's a myriad of ways that the unhealthily frugal energy of the Four of Pentacles could show up for you as an individual, so that's why doing a tarot spread about this card will help gain clarity on what it is exactly that you're being too (mentally or monetarily) stingy about.

This point in the Minor Arcana and in pregnancy might be when we might start hearing the call beckoning us to connect our decisions for the future with our societal impact. You might be thinking about possibly cloth diapering but squashing the idea before you give it a fair shot because you think it will be too hard. You might be feeling called to do the inner shadow work of ending the ancestral cycles of trauma, abuse, racism, and so on so that you don't pass that on to your baby/legacy, but maybe you're dismissing the idea of a therapist or antiracism educator as too expensive before researching to see if any offer services on a sliding scale.

If you feel yourself avoiding something, that is a sign to be curious about it and dive in deeper. You can make the difficult but morally right choice here, whatever that may be for you. The universe will have your back if you do.

◁ FOUR OF PENTACLES THEMES ▷

generosity, investing in your birth team from a place of integrity, healing scarcity mindset, introspection, deciding what you're going to be ethically rooted in as a parent

TAROT SPREAD FOR HONING INTUITION AND REMOVING SELF-LIMITING BLOCKAGES

What is one tool I have available to me that I don't utilize enough?

What brain blockage is telling me a story that is holding me back?

What energy will help me connect with my intuition with more depth and clarity?

What is a message my intuition/ancestors/Spirit/guides have for me right now?

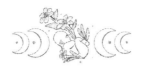

THE FIVES

"You do not have to be fearless to birth in total power. Recognizing and working with our fears is how we learn to distinguish them from our intuition."

—Jonea Cunico RN, childbirth educator*

❧ MONTH 5 THEMES ☙

transitioning from the first half of pregnancy to the second half of pregnancy (transitions are rarely easy), beginning to feel fear of birth and postpartum now that the meaning of "halfway there" is setting in, beginning to get caught up in negative beliefs or negative expectations about birth or postpartum, feeling trapped or as though there's no going back

IN THE PHYSICAL BODY

Your fetus is about the size of a banana right now—halfway there! They can also hear better now (including the sounds in your environment, not only your heartbeat and voice anymore) and they can now also detect light outside your belly.

Estrogen levels are high right now, which account for some intensity of moods, but it might also make you feel particularly fluid and sensual. This is a common time

----

* Find Jonea Cunico online at Wild Pregnancy Free Birth (wpfbeducation.com) and @wild.pregnancy _free.birth.

to start feeling acid reflux and heartburn. The hormone relaxin that's helping your body prepare to make space for a growing fetus is also causing the muscles in your esophagus to relax (which causes the heartburn) and slows your digestion (causing gas or constipation).

Similar to nausea, a way to mitigate these digestive ailments is to eat smaller, more frequent meals throughout the day instead of a few larger meals. Probiotics help with this too.

FIVE OF CUPS

In the Fives, we are transitioning from the first half of pregnancy to the latter half, and transitions are notoriously strenuous, physically and emotionally. Nearly every Five has a bit of a bitter taste to it, and the Five of Cups is no exception. This card is often characterized by sadness induced by disappointment or lingering sadness from a previous grief rupture. Perhaps you learned that your best friend who you wanted to care for you postpartum will be out of town at the time. Perhaps you got a gestational diabetes diagnosis. Perhaps you're having a hard time setting boundaries with your family or your partner's family, and it's taking a toll on your mental health, and you can't help catastrophizing and worrying how this will manifest once the baby is here. Whatever the scenario is, you're in your feelings right now, not yet searching for the silver lining, and for now, that's okay. Over half your cups of expectations are knocked over and empty, and that does suck, but some are still upright.

As always, let yourself feel your feelings, but be warned not to give in entirely to defeat or self-pity here. There is always autonomy to be found in a situation, even when the landscape of your situation isn't ideal, even when you have to let go of your ideal expectation.

Yes, at best, something is disappointing; at worst, something is actually lost. But this card has a very mental energy for the normally emotional suit of the cups. The water in this card is showing up in the form of clouds, muddying our perception of reality. Mourn what you need to and feel your feelings, but remember to stay grounded in reality, the tangible facts of what did or didn't happen. And if you can't sift your way through these mental clouds, at least make sure you're not making decisions from this place, in this moment. Vital decisions can wait until the fog has cleared.

⤳ FIVE OF CUPS THEMES ⤶

*halfway there, depression, transitions, catastrophizing circumstances,
disappointment, being emotionally down and having a hard time getting out of it,
being too "in your head," call in your resources for accountability and reflection*

FIVE OF WANDS

Halfway through pregnancy has some gravity to it, doesn't it? It's normal to have a moment of fear or panic at the no-going-back nature of this halfway point, and sometimes this manifests as irritability or resistance against transition. You might be looking to pick a fight with your partner, your older children, or anyone who crosses your path because you're agitated and don't quite know why.

Pause.

Allow yourself the vulnerability of seeing that at the root of your resistance is fear of shit getting real. This card is quintessential *Well, if I'm struggling so badly with XYZ right now, what am I going to do when the baby is actually here?!* energy.

This card is another great lesson for birth. Transition during labor—the transition from active labor to the pushing phase where the cervix is no longer just expanding, babe is descending, and the body is taking over to eject the baby—is often met with fear, wanting to give up, and a sense of erratic flailing, physically and/or mentally. In labor, this is often the point when birthing people say they "can't do it" or ask for pain medication.

We need to be held, contained, and reassured that it's almost over during transitions. We need to be given the space and vulnerability to not fight it anymore, but to expand, even if it's scary to release and let go of our grip so we can bloom into that expansion. Birthing folks need to feel safe being vulnerable, knowing that their vulnerability and fear won't be translated into disempowerment or unwanted intervention, no matter what kind of birth they're choosing or experiencing.

So, if you're experiencing this energy at the halfway point in your pregnancy, then it might just be a trial run for the intensity and out-of-control feelings that can come with labor.

⤳ FIVES OF WANDS THEMES ⤶

*halfway there and maybe freaking out a little, unhealthy comparison, feeling out of
control, practice for labor, resistance to change or loss, feeling defeated*

FIVE OF SWORDS

Coinciding with the energies at play in the Five of Wands—fear, flailing, fighting—you might also be experiencing negative self-talk. Halfway there, labor, birth, and post-partum can either be a beacon to the future or an ominous, looming eventuality, and the Five of Swords deals with the latter.

After resting in the Four of Swords, you've picked your arms back up again and are ready for a fight. It's worth pausing to consider whether this fight is a worthy one or not (or maybe if now is just not the right time for that fight). Postpone potential confrontation for a week or two and see how you feel then. Don't make decisions for the future from this offensive state.

Earlier decisions you made in your pregnancy might start to feel scary to carry out now that birth is more tangibly on your horizon. Many people will want to sow seeds of doubt that disempower you and make you feel like you can't do it . . . but don't let one of those voices of doubt be your own.

This card points out that you might be your own worst enemy (not just in pregnancy, but likely in a cycle that's shown up in other ways in your life), so doing the work now to end that self-destructive cycle will be what gets you through the transition.

ᕤ FIVE OF SWORDS THEMES ᕗ

halfway there and grasping for control, fighting a fight we don't have to be fighting, sacrificing your own peace to be right, over-worrying about the future, defensiveness, what you need might be found in precisely what you resist, not knowing what's next

FIVE OF PENTACLES

This card is traditionally interpreted as financial destitution, but it can speak to scarcity in all forms and resources, especially the feeling of scarcity that occurs when you don't feel connected with your intuition or magical gifts.

This shows up as knowing you need help but feeling the self-punitive need to suffer alone without reaching out. Or getting in a funk and falling off doing whatever rituals helped you feel connected to the divine, so you feel as though your inner voice is muddied.

If it helps, this notion that our lack of resources is only ours to bear without ever allowing our community to witness or show up for us in that is also a nasty by-product of the capitalist, white-supremacist culture that we are all currently steeped in and have been steeped in for the last several centuries.

The idea of "pulling yourself up by your bootstraps" is a cruel and violent notion for folks who were never given the privilege of boots in the first place. The sense of isolation and financial destitution that this card invokes is exactly what white supremacy culture wants you to feel—as if it's your own fault that you don't have the resources that all humans deserve. White supremacy culture wants you disconnected from your divine ancestral support and intuitive lifeline, because it's easier to coerce and sell things to people who feel lost, disconnected, and underresourced. To admit that it is the capitalist, white-supremacist patriarchy that is responsible for your lack and that the legacy and culture of bootstrapism* is a cruel and inhumane outlook on life would be white supremacy shooting itself in its own dirty boot.

Now that we've debunked the idea that you're not deserving of basic human needs and reminded you that you are divine no matter how "connected" or "disconnected" to your intuition you feel at this moment, how do we move forward and take the next step in this when it still feels as if there won't be enough for us? How do we keep going when we fear that we won't be supported, or the resources we need to feel secure are nowhere in visible sight?

We pause—for as long as we need to, with trust, until the next right step ahead materializes for us. We assess if we *need* to take a step forward at this moment, or if it can wait a breath, a day, a week, a month, until we're no longer feeling panic about not having what we need (either support, resources, safety, or otherwise). And if the next step never arrives, we ask for help. Reaching out through the barrier of isolation and feeling deserving of leaning on your community is revolutionary.

Halfway there is still a long way to go. It may not feel like there is an abundance of resources for you but there is an abundance of time (relatively). So, take your time.

ᐛ FIVE OF PENTACLES THEMES ᕫ

halfway there but still a long way to go, being worthy of rest, being worthy of being taken care of, rewriting ancestral scripts around productivity, scarcity of resources, trusting what's next

. . . .

* Again, understanding how "pulling yourself up by your bootstraps" is a consequence of privilege can be credited to leaders in the world of antiracism such as educator Rachel Cargle, and her pivotal work on Patreon, *The Great Unlearn*.

HERBAL TEA
FOR HEARTBURN AND DIGESTION

The marshmallow root coats the lining of the esophagus and stomach, which has been found effective in reducing the sensations of heartburn (this can make it contraindicated if you're on any medications that it might prevent from being absorbed, so consult your care provider). The ginger helps aid digestion and alleviate any nausea that may accompany the heartburn. The peppermint soothes the immediate discomfort of heartburn.

INGREDIENTS

2 tsp peppermint leaf

1 tsp dried or fresh ginger

1 tsp marshmallow root

DIRECTIONS

Add all the ingredients to a tea strainer and steep in a mug of hot water for 3 to 5 minutes. Sweeten to taste if you prefer.

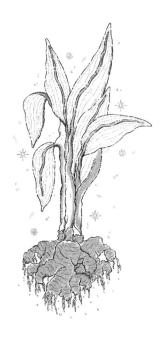

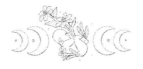

THE SIXES

❧ MONTH 6 THEMES ❧

overcoming the discomfort of the transition in the Fives by focusing on health and nutrition; controlling what you can control; having a spiritual breakthrough; delving into residual necessary shadow work that will otherwise surface during your birth, postpartum, and parenting experiences; a good time to reclaim your sexuality in your changing physical body; being objective; a good time to begin writing your birth preferences and plans; a return of joy and excited anticipation after a pessimistic fifth month

IN THE PHYSICAL BODY

Your fetus is putting on fat finally, so they're the size of a big plump papaya right now. This is the last month of your second trimester, and this is when you might start to feel "big," meaning that lower back pain can intensify in this month. So, if you're not already seeing a chiropractor or doing the exercises we talked about in month 4, there's no time like the present!

SIX OF CUPS

The energy of this card is a call to reclaim your sense of being grounded, control, and joy in your life through the vehicle of coming home to your sexuality. The Sixes are another sturdy and balanced number. So, if things feel surprisingly good right now, just like the Four of Wands, don't question it, don't fight it, let good be good, and use this time to utilize that good in order to do the things your nauseated, cranky, first-trimester self wasn't up for.

This card is similar to and connected to the energy of the Strength card, so you might want to visit that chapter in the Major Arcana section (page 189).

If you're someone who is open to utilizing magical, intentional sex with yourself or your partner, it would be a good time to tap into that resource for the purpose of doing inner-child-healing or ancestral-healing work, if that feels safe and accessible for you to do. The vulnerabilities opened and potential energy heightened during sex and orgasm is a potent addition to any spell work, but it is particularly useful for healing traumas that have set up shop within your body. Usually if this card comes up, and at this point in pregnancy, you're in a place that can handle that kind of heavy right now. But as always, tap in and make sure that it is aligned.

Revisit the things you shove down, what keeps you dwelling in shame, bring it to the surface, and then intentionally release it. Identify what your tea was steeped in, whether toxic or healthy. That is, what cultural conditioning, internalized supremacy, internalized misogyny, internalized unworthiness, abusive tendencies, and the like were you raised with that you don't want to carry forth when you are a parent yourself?

⊰ SIX OF CUPS THEMES ⊱

coming back home to the sexual self, a joyful pause, feeling good in your body again, sex as an intentional vehicle for healing, assessing your conditioning around modesty and purity culture

ƎXERCISE

DETOXIFYING CLEANSE

If what you uncover in this work is toxic, do a detoxifying herbal bath or take an intentionally energetic cleansing shower. Visualize the sludge you were steeped in escaping through your pores, out of your body, out of your sphere of influence, at least for now. This is a regular practice, not a one-time thing. If you are taking a shower, imagine the toxicity of your upbringing escaping through your pores until you are emptied. Then, draw yourself a bath, fill it with herbs of goodness, love, manifestation, and protection. Allow your now-emptied self to absorb all that goodness instead, allow it to soften in the new, welcoming warmth of this environment. A great way to signify or intensify the feeling of release after a cleansing ritual such as this is to have an orgasm (preferably one where you are vocal and taking up whatever space you need), if that is something that is accessible or desirable to you.

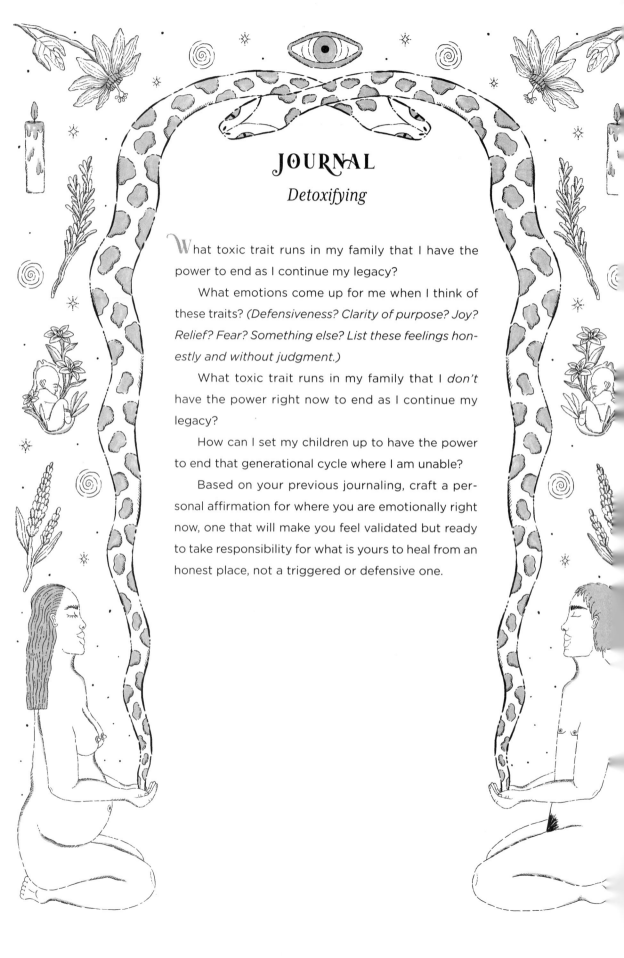

JOURNAL

Detoxifying

What toxic trait runs in my family that I have the power to end as I continue my legacy?

What emotions come up for me when I think of these traits? *(Defensiveness? Clarity of purpose? Joy? Relief? Fear? Something else? List these feelings honestly and without judgment.)*

What toxic trait runs in my family that I *don't* have the power right now to end as I continue my legacy?

How can I set my children up to have the power to end that generational cycle where I am unable?

Based on your previous journaling, craft a personal affirmation for where you are emotionally right now, one that will make you feel validated but ready to take responsibility for what is yours to heal from an honest place, not a triggered or defensive one.

SIX OF WANDS

You've made it this far, and you're probably feeling very pregnant! And it's beautiful, no matter what your body type or how your baby bump is shaping up. Your womb's creative art project might be starting to be more visible to the world, and it's normal to want to show it off. If you feel this urge, follow it. Take some sensual selfies of you and your bump, or if you have the resources available to you, hire a photographer for a boudoir maternity shoot, whichever you're more comfortable with or whatever aligns with your goals for how you want to feel right now.

You don't have to share them with anybody if you don't want to; this is just a way to document this part in your journey toward parenthood and honor where you are and the big, beautiful work your body is doing.

Allow whatever art you make right now—photographic or otherwise—to be true, real, and raw representations of the inner landscape of your creativity, sensuality, and whatever else lights you up. This isn't the kind of self-art that has the gaze of others in mind at all (though if you choose to share your self-art, that's your business!). Let this be as messy, authentic, opulent, or extravagant as you want.

We all deserve to see ourselves represented in such a venerated light, pregnant or not. Humans are expressions of divinity, and making another human is an extension of that expression, so try to let your unfiltered inner voice have the mic more than the voice of self-doubt or self-consciousness.

⤙ SIX OF WANDS THEMES ⤚

creative expression, creativity as a path to understanding intuition, mind/body connection, enjoying some peace after the difficulty of the Fives, self-worship, confidence

SIX OF SWORDS

This card indicates leaving behind what so absolutely, undeniably, and without a doubt needs to be left behind. If you hired an OB, a midwife, a doula, or if you have a partner and it's just not jiving, you're not respected, or you're not heard, then it's time to go. Scary as that may be, the longer you wait, the harder it will become (and expect to be revisited by this energy in the eighth month if you don't address it now).

As inconvenient as it is to have to walk away from something you've already invested time or energy or even money into, you're robbing yourself of the possibility of how *good* it feels to be in communion with a birth team or a partner that is totally aligned with your energy and needs. You deserve walking away. Trust that something else is possible. Because something else *is* possible.

While letting go and leaving shit behind is undoubtedly the message of this card, that is not necessarily accessible for everyone. If you feel you're in relationship with someone or something that is truly not aligned, and you explored every possible avenue for disengagement and still find it to be an impossibility, there are other ways to honor this energy when it's asking for your attention. Use the journal prompts from the Six of Cups (page 76) to unlearn stale, old thought patterns, to release ancestral baggage, and to engage journaling, breath work, and other healing modalities. There is something accessible to everyone, as a means of physically, mentally, or energetically letting something go. Utilize a waning moon period to assist you in whatever you're shedding.

◁ SIX OF SWORDS THEMES ▷

ending relationships with anyone in your life, letting go, shedding ancestral baggage, seeking what's more aligned by first leaving behind what's not working

SIX OF PENTACLES

One way to let something go is to give it away to someone else. I know there's plenty of things we need to walk away from that we can't tangibly give to someone else, so this can also mean giving it up to the universe, your ancestors, or guides to take care of it for you.

Or if you're someone who is living from a place of resource abundance right now, try practicing abundance magic by giving some of what you have away by setting up a regular practice of mutual aid. This signals to the universe that you trust there will always be enough for you. Also, allow yourself to receive and accept blessings as readily as you'd be generous with others, because you're worthy of the generosity of others and the benevolence of the universe too.

Given the history of birth covered later in this book by Stephanie Mitchell about how the field of midwifery was colonized and how that still affects birthing folks today, one of the most abundantly multiplying places you can share your resources is funding Black and Indigenous student midwives. Because of colonization, there aren't enough of them to meet the needs of their communities. The work they do is at the very root of life and their impact has a multiplication effect on the families they serve. This makes funding Black and Indigenous midwives my preferred mode of abundance magic spending and regular reparation* payments.

⊰ SIX OF PENTACLES THEMES ⊱

generosity, abundance, having enough, money magic, delegating, giving problems away to the ancestors to deal with on your behalf

. . . .

* Reparations are owed from folks who have colonizer ancestry to folks who have been colonized because we (speaking for myself as a person who has colonizer ancestry) were able to build our generational wealth off unpaid labor for kidnapped, trafficked, and enslaved African people, on land that was stolen from the people who are Indigenous to Turtle Island (which refers to what is now called the continent of North America). Reparations were owed at the time of emancipation for the life and labor stolen, but those attempts at paying reparations were always interrupted by the systems and people upholding white supremacy. To that end, they have never been paid, resulting in generational inequities, so it is up to us to pay reparations on behalf of our ancestors as a generational debt owed. Again, educational content on reparations is not something I can claim credit for, but rather credit is due to antiracism educators and activists who have been fighting for government-level reparations for decades.

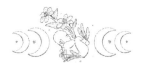

THE SEVENS

◁ MONTH 7 THEMES ▷

*confusion; a reprise of negative expectations due to the presentation of new obstacles;
now that we've written down how we would prefer our birth to go, there is something
to lose, there is a more tangible option for "failure"; now that we've written down our
birth preferences, there is more opportunity for outside opinion to interfere with our
resolve; setting boundaries; our self-knowledge and intuition is being tested here, so it
will be time to take a stand and hold fast to our truths*

IN THE PHYSICAL BODY

Month 7 is where you shift into the third trimester! Your fetus is likely starting to get
a little cramped in there now that they are about as long as they'll be when they're
born. From here on out, they're adding on fat and maturing their lungs. At this point
in pregnancy, it's also not uncommon for you to experience leg cramps, restless legs,
or itchiness, and magnesium is your friend for these symptoms. The herbal infusion
on page 55 (which I know you're diligently, regularly drinking, riiiight?) is high in
magnesium, so that will help, but eating lots of watermelon or taking magnesium
supplements can help too.

SEVEN OF CUPS

There is a reprise of the difficulty and confusion of the Five of Cups, except this time,
you have the opportunity to transmute fear and uncertainty into an almost childlike

curiosity. Think of the wonder that can be induced by psychedelics, and you'll know the energy of this card. What if we approached the problems in our pregnancy from that same place of curiosity and wonder? In this way, the card is another teacher for preparing for labor and birth.

If you're someone who has ever used psychoactive drugs, you know that fear is a recipe for a bad trip. Trying to resist their influence, and the journey on which the drugs want to take you, will most surely make for a less desirable experience. It's often in bravely opening yourself and stepping fully into the fear that you can be in curious wonder of the entirely new experience your body is undergoing.

Experiences like this, whether it be DMT produced naturally by your pineal gland during birth, or drugs/plant medicine explored during your experimental prepregnancy days, are opportunities to observe our souls trying to strip down to their essence. Ego is not necessarily a good or bad thing, but our soul is not defined by it, and experiences like birth and other psychedelic trips require us to surrender the ego to these cosmic experiences with wonder and awe. Fear can definitely play a vital, informative role in our journey to expansion and transformation, but it is meant to be an obstacle, not a roadblock.

This isn't the brain or the ego's time to shine (those things get their say in many other energies of the tarot); this is a time to make a soul-centered emotional exploration of your inner world. Start preparing for the otherworldly possibilities that might come to you during labor and utilize that mystery to get excited about the cosmic journey of birth.

ᕤ SEVEN OF CUPS THEMES ᕬ

adopting a childlike curiosity about your hard problems, feeling your way
through difficulty, psychedelic experiences during labor, enlightenment,
cosmic pregnancy and birth

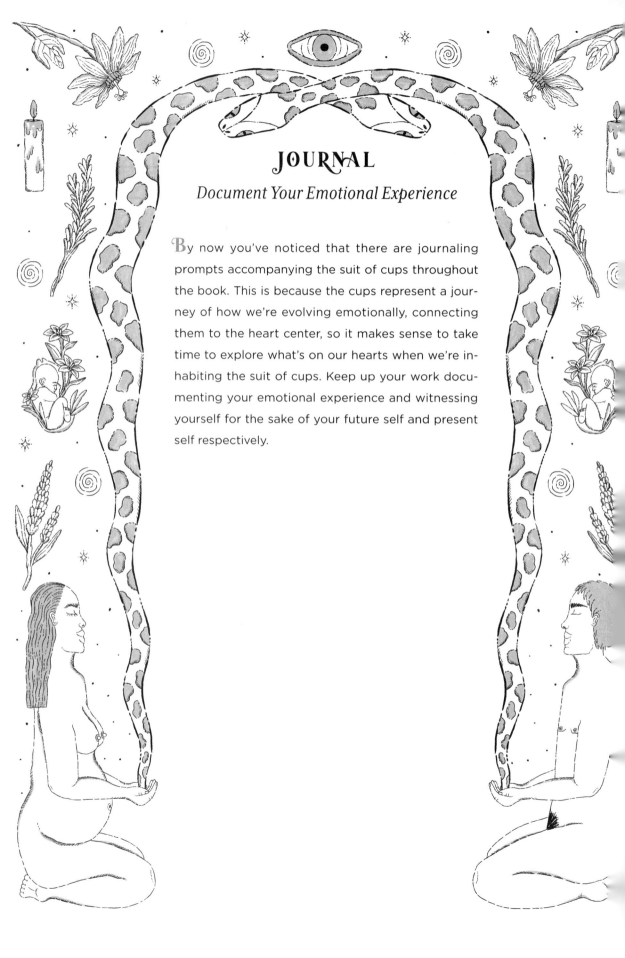

JOURNAL

Document Your Emotional Experience

By now you've noticed that there are journaling prompts accompanying the suit of cups throughout the book. This is because the cups represent a journey of how we're evolving emotionally, connecting them to the heart center, so it makes sense to take time to explore what's on our hearts when we're inhabiting the suit of cups. Keep up your work documenting your emotional experience and witnessing yourself for the sake of your future self and present self respectively.

SEVEN OF WANDS

It can be disempowering to feel misunderstood or dismissed. The energy of this card speaks to expecting that kind of fight or misunderstanding, and it may or may not be rooted in reality.

By now, you likely have a solid birth plan in place, the kind you feel good about (if you don't, visit the Emperor chapter in the Major Arcana section, page 178). But that also means people may start to ask about those plans. And if you've chosen anything other than standard hospital care and doing whatever the doctor says, especially if you've made some choices or plans that are culturally unpopular, don't expect that folks will be willing or open to learn about all the time, intuition, and research you put into making your choices. Humbly curious people do exist, and I hope they're in your orbit, but they are unfortunately few and far between. If you're making alternative birth choices of any kind, expect covert or overt judgment. If you are expecting to be judged, I understand why, but in the Seven of Wands, it's important not to assume or project what people are thinking and stay open to conversations unfolding.

You can trust yourself to stay rooted in your research and plans, even if the people you're conversing with about your pregnancy and birth are less than supportive of your choices.

I'm giving you permission, right now, to take any judgmental side-eye or awkward pause offered in response to anything you share with people about your birth plan as a free pass to set up a boundary with that person. It doesn't have to be forever; it doesn't have to be such a rock-solid boundary that you cut them out of your life entirely (unless that's what you feel is called for). The Seven of Wands calls for establishing boundaries to keep people at un-intimate distances. People will show you who they are in their actions and reactions, whether they will be judgmental or supportive. Believe them when they show you who they are and how they plan to respect (or not respect) your choices. These kinds of relationships can muddy your intuition and your peace of mind, so it's okay to put a light pause on this relationship until you no longer feel judgment coming from them.

◁ SEVEN OF WANDS THEMES ▷

conflict, feeling like you must prove yourself, other people's judgments,
projections, harmful comparison, unsolicited advice, disagreements with
your care provider, self-trust

SEVEN OF SWORDS

The Seven of Swords goes hand in hand with the Seven of Wands, though the energy of this card represents when we've let people's judgment and negative expectations for us seep into our psyche. In turn, we start to be ruled by those voices in our head—and not our own voice.

Having a concrete birth plan and hopes and dreams for your birth and your baby means we now have something to lose. Now that things are more decided, the interfering opinions of others can often flow in, unwarranted and unwanted, and they might hold more weight than they normally would because of any possible fear we may be carrying about having something to lose.

This card is a call to get back to the center. Strip away anything clinging to you that is not yours.

⊰ SEVEN OF SWORDS THEMES ⊱
allowing people to get under your skin, doubt, projections,
coming back to center, boundaries

EXERCISE

CLEARING YOUR INTUITION
FROM DOUBTFUL VOICES

Here is an exercise for clearing out doubtful voices that are not your intuition: On one sheet of paper, write the title "Doubtful Voices," and on a second sheet, title the page "My Internal Voice." Consider all the negative or doubtful things floating around in your mind right now. Then put them into categories. Does this thing come from your own wondering? If so, write that concern on the sheet titled "My Internal Voice." Or does this thing come from some kind of doubtful input projected onto you? Keep in mind, it's not just people directly placing doubt on your choices around pregnancy, birth, and parenting that can muddy your internal dialogue—media you've viewed or other people's experiences you've passively learned about are also things that cling to you. Write these external doubts on the sheet titled "Doubtful Voices."

If there is anything you listed as coming from your own internal voice without any outside influence, then save that page of concerns to discuss with your midwife, doctor, or doula. Worries are lessened when they are shared, and their power is diffused when spoken out loud in the light of day instead of just clanging around in your head, building pressure.

Then, take those worries that you listed as projections of other folks' doubts, bad experiences, or media input. Using a fire-safe bowl or cauldron, burn the paper, watching intentionally how their ill-intended words get eaten up by the fire. Notice how frail the paper and words are once they've become ash, how they dissolve with the slightest touch or puff of air. (*Always be careful whenever you are doing a ceremony or ritual involving fire. It is a powerful element and one we need to engage with cautiously and respectfully.*)

Remember: That same fire, the same ability to burn up ill intentions, exists in you. It is always available to you when someone tries to diminish the bright flame of your truth. Stay true to the values from which you have made your choices. Tune out the noise trying to sow doubt or fear. You're smart enough to know the difference between good advice that's just hard to hear and fear-based advice that's possibly rooted in the advice-giver's own trauma and projection. Use your discernment. Stay focused on what you know to be true for you and your baby. Only you know that. Call upon the energy of the Seven of Wands to help you set whatever boundaries you need.

SEVEN OF PENTACLES

Month 7 is a good time to get your house in order. It's not as fun as picking out cute baby clothes for your registry, but you are being called to handle the brass tacks of baby rearing, health insurance, finalizing payments, and more. The work you do now will be what sets you up for a transition into parenthood that's as easy as it can be.

It's the time in your pregnancy to do the boring stuff you've neglected to do until now, such as doing your taxes, finally starting to see a chiropractor, taking a birth class with your partner, or reading that one book. This card is about "doing the work," specifically, the less fun, but still important work.

Revisit any previous chapter that you felt uncomfortable or avoidant reading. Notice if you still feel uncomfortable in that energy, or if it's not as provoking now that you've learned more.

Now, revisit any previous chapter you skipped over, putting it off as work for a "rainy day." The Seven of Pentacles says today is that "rainy day." Be thorough. Don't skip any steps. Whether you're doing your inner-child or ancestral healing, don't leave stones unturned just because you want to avoid what you might discover.

You signed up for continuing your family legacy when you decided to become a parent. In hearing those words, how do they sit? Is it a family legacy you're proud of and want to perpetuate? If not, it's time to get to work in ensuring that what you're passing down is intentional. If you're not sure where to start in that work, pull another card to guide you, or visit page 158 where resources for deeper learning and ancestral healing are shared.

⊰ SEVEN OF PENTACLES THEMES ⊱

tending to our environment, being thorough, setting yourself up for success, the brass tacks not-so-fun-part of becoming a parent, "doing the work"

SOOTHING BELLY RUB

As your belly begins to stretch, it's not uncommon for you to experience itchiness on your belly. So, whether or not you're concerned about stretch marks, it's still a good idea to keep the skin of your belly hydrated and supple to prevent itchiness and promote flexibility.

Like most of the recipes I share, every ingredient plays a different part in the recipe, but don't be discouraged and not make anything at all just because you might not have all the ingredients listed. Something is better than nothing! You could rub your belly with nothing but coconut oil for your whole pregnancy, and that would do the trick; this recipe just has a few more skin-nourishing and stretch-promoting properties to it.

INGREDIENTS

Dried plantain leaf (see Note)
Jojoba oil (or any other carrier oil such as olive oil or avocado oil)
½ cup coconut oil
Beeswax (optional, for a firmer body butter)
20 to 30 drops vitamin E oil (optional)
Essential oils (optional)

DIRECTIONS

First, you must first infuse your carrier oil with the dried plantain leaf. Place the plantain leaf in a glass jar and cover it completely with the jojoba oil, ensuring no leaves are exposed to air. Let sit for 4 to 6 weeks to infuse, shaking periodically. Alternatively, you can do a fast infusion by placing this jar (with the lid on) in a crockpot with 1 or 2 inches of water in the bottom, with a small towel at the bottom to act as a buffer between the glass jar and the crockpot so the glass jar doesn't crack. This method will very slowly heat the oil. Allow it to infuse on low heat for 12 to 24 hours. Whether you choose the long or quick infusion, once it is finished, strain out the leaves with a strainer or cheesecloth. This oil is now ready for you to use for this recipe, and anything else you'd like to add it to.

In a stainless steel or glass pot, gently melt your coconut oil (and beeswax if you want more of a salve texture). Do not ever let this mixture get to the point of smoking or boiling. You're just trying to heat the ingredients enough to melt them. Once fully melted, turn off the heat, and add 1 Tbsp of the plantain oil and the vitamin E oil. At this point, you may add any other essential oils for aromatherapy purposes, if desired.

Pour the oil mixture into a glass container and allow it to cool completely before putting on the lid. From there, you can store it at room temperature. As you apply it, give your belly/baby a massage, feeling where your baby is and giving some love to your internal organs for how hard they're working for you. Use this ritual as an opportunity to get quiet and connect with your wombmate.

I would apply this twice a day, in the morning upon getting out of the shower, and before bed. If you didn't add in essential oils to your recipe, you can repurpose anything you have left as a nipple balm or diaper rash salve during postpartum.

NOTE: Plantain leaf is a plant that most folks on Turtle Island (the so-called United States) would consider a weed, except for those who know its potent healing medicine. In the summer in much of North America, plantain leaf grows wild. This is important because if buying herbs is not accessible for you, it's likely that this incredibly useful plant is available for free right under your feet, in the cracks of the sidewalk. It is healing and soothing for irritated skin, scars, burns, diaper rash, eczema, and perineal tears, so you can see why this plant ally wants to be your friend during pregnancy, postpartum, and parenthood.

In order to be able to use plantain leaf, first confirm that what you're picking is actually plantain leaf and choose plants from an area that doesn't get a lot of foot traffic. Ask the plants if they are okay with coming home with you to be made into medicine and offer gratitude and reciprocity however you choose. Gather as much as you need to fill your preferred glass container, and then a little more (as plantain leaves shrink as they dry). Wash them very well (plantain grows low to the ground, so there will be dirt!), and then lay them out to dry somewhere well ventilated on a paper towel or cooling rack. Allow 3 to 4 days for complete drying. You now have a very potent medicine that can be used in a myriad of ways for tending to your own body and your future kiddo's body that cost you nothing but your time.

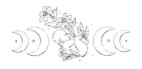

THE EIGHTS

❧ MONTH 8 THEMES ❧

*beginning to release; communication; continuing to work through the murky
confusion of the Sevens but this time with more urgency; time to finalize decisions;
selective use of time, energy, and resources*

IN THE PHYSICAL BODY

At eight months, your fetus is developing and practicing all the things they will need for digestion outside your uterus, practicing more swallowing, sucking, and breathing amniotic fluid, as the digestive system prepares to transition from being nourished only by the placenta to being nourished via their mouth. It's not uncommon for Braxton-Hicks* contractions to occur at this point (if not even earlier), especially after vigorous activity, sex, or something bumping into your belly. These

---

* Braxton-Hicks contractions are named after an English obstetrician who first named the contractions that occur earlier in pregnancy that don't result in birth. But this bodily function played a role in preparing for birth long before a cisgendered man came along to name and claim it, so this function ought to be named after the brilliance of the body, not after the man who observed it and decided to name it. These are sometimes called "practice contractions" or "false labor"—but there is nothing false about them! They are how your uterus tones itself in preparation for labor, and they are not concerning at this point unless they become intense or consistently spaced and close together. They feel like menstrual cramps, though some people don't feel them at all and rather feel the sensation or tightening of their bellies. If you're feeling as though your preparation contractions are too close together or intense, the reason for this can be dehydration, so drink plenty of fluids (preferably water with a pinch of salt, or bone broth), take a rest on your left side, and reduce whatever activity has triggered them.

early contractions not only prepare your uterus for the contractions of labor, but they also protect your fetus.

Your pregnancy guidebook or app will inform you about every possible weird symptom you might have at this point, and leading up to it. I have the anecdotal opinion that pregnancy symptoms all have a purpose: forgetfulness is a reminder to do less (maybe you didn't really *need* to remember that thing), and so your body decided to discard that information taking up space in your brain. Blurry vision might be preparing us to see the world from our baby's perspective once they're earthside. Low or high blood sugar is a sign your nutrition needs attention and near-constant tending, much like your baby will need near-constant nutritional intake after they're born. High blood pressure can be a call to remove stressors from your life so those stressful energies are not present once you are postpartum and your baby can be influenced by those energies. Your "overly sensitive" mood is mimicking how sensitive your newborn's experience of the world will be, and preparing you to understand their experience. Heartburn is a call to rest and be slow and intentional about your nutritional intake. Your areolas darken so your newborn, who won't have very good vision at the time of birth, will more easily see and find them.

The list goes on, so I invite you to take your weirdest, most seemingly pointless pregnancy symptom, and dig into research or meditate on what that symptom is trying to teach you. None of that is to suggest avoiding consulting with your care provider if you're experiencing any of these ailments, because they may be indicative of health issues that need to be addressed and possibly managed. But no matter their severity, I do not believe that the long list of pregnancy symptoms is just random, annoying, or without purpose.

EIGHT OF CUPS

You know that thing that the Six of Swords (and your intuition) was telling you that you need to walk away from in your sixth month of pregnancy (see page 77)? Well, if you didn't address it then, the Eight of Cups is dragging it back up, and this time the message is even louder, clearer, and likely a little bit more difficult or painful to walk away from given that it's been dragged out longer and further attachments and entanglements have formed in the last two months. In fact, all the Eights are going to be in dealing with this situation, and they will each be an ally in helping you through the difficulty that is letting go.

Traditionally this card looks like a person walking away from eight upright cups, indicating that time and effort was invested. But the message of this card is clear: There is nothing more for you here. No matter how much you invested in it, it's time to go. Whether it's a professional you hired, a partner, an unhealthy habit, a friendship, or a toxic or limiting way of thinking about yourself or your pregnancy, you likely already know what it is you need to let go of and walk away from without looking back, and here is the chance to do so.

Here, directness and clarity of intention is going to be favored over beating around the bush. Compassionate, resolute firmness is going to be favored over manipulation and game playing. Vulnerability is going to be favored over defensiveness. Choose to stand on the favored side with trust that you are divinely cared for (because you are!). And use gentle care with yourself as you recover from any wounds this departure might have left with you.

⪥ EIGHT OF CUPS THEMES ⪤

walking away once and for all, messages being louder, breaking off ties with someone, leaving behind an old way of being, endings with accountability and right relationship

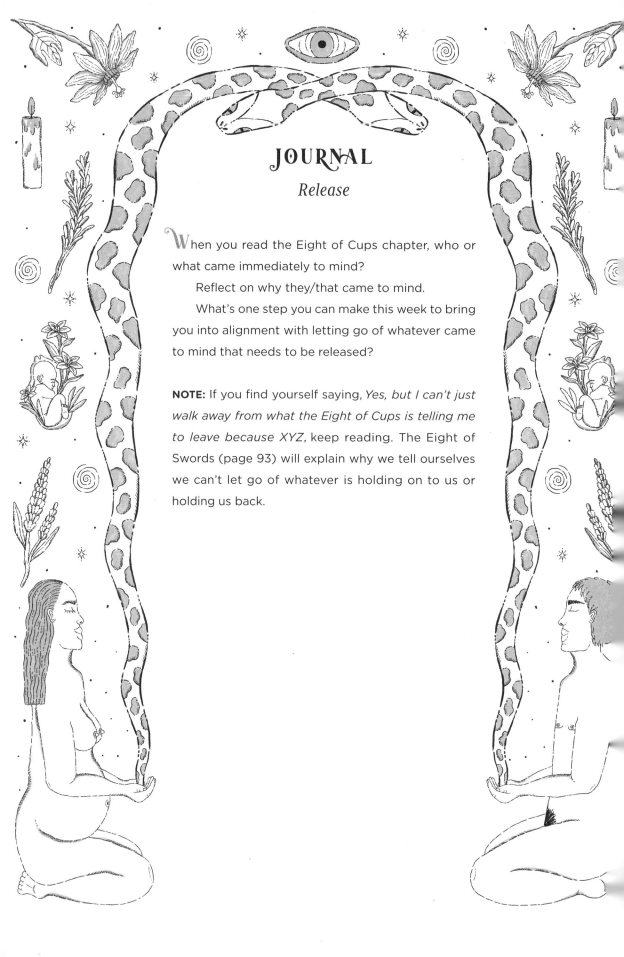

JOURNAL

Release

When you read the Eight of Cups chapter, who or what came immediately to mind?

Reflect on why they/that came to mind.

What's one step you can make this week to bring you into alignment with letting go of whatever came to mind that needs to be released?

NOTE: If you find yourself saying, *Yes, but I can't just walk away from what the Eight of Cups is telling me to leave because XYZ*, keep reading. The Eight of Swords (page 93) will explain why we tell ourselves we can't let go of whatever is holding on to us or holding us back.

EIGHT OF SWORDS

The Eight of Swords takes the situation or person that we know we need to walk away from and injects it with a good dose of fear. You might panic and feel as if even though you're clear on what you need to do, there is no way out. Maybe you're caught up and entangled in a story that's not actually rooted in reality or your truth. Maybe you're too invested, too cautious, or too afraid.

But, of course, there is always some way out (even if that doesn't look as clean as you'd like). The Eight of Swords, however, is speaking specifically to the brain chemistry that wants to convince you that there is no escape. This card cautions you against being ruled by that paranoid, fearful brain chemistry.

And yet, this card is still an ally. It is not pushing you through or forcing you to get over your fears. Rather, the medicine of this card is a pause. You don't have to decide to walk away from what entangles you right this second. You don't even have to do it tomorrow or the next day. Go slow.

Allow your brain to have its say as it speaks for its fear and anxieties, and then go inward (meditate, move your body, journal, pull cards, stare at a candle, watch the sunrise) to soothe your soul and nervous system. You can move forward once the acuity of the fear has passed and it is no longer the loudest voice you're hearing.

ᛡ EIGHT OF SWORDS THEMES ᛣ
feeling trapped by your circumstances, your fears as a communicator, caution against feeling defeated before trying, don't rush big decisions

EIGHT OF WANDS

The Eight of Wands arrives to directly aid in the clear, calm, vulnerable communication needed to carry out the task, offering the courage we feel we lack in the Eight of Swords.

This card is shedding light on all the confusion and darkness, which makes it much simpler to see the situation with clarity and objectivity. The Eight of Wands is an ally in helping us be less emotionally bound to the situation. Things can be more clear-cut now, and a path forward is visible where it once was not.

The direct communication that the Eight of Cups asks of us is bolstered by this card. So, if the reason you haven't left what you know you need to leave behind is that you're anxious about how it will go, take heart. Carry the image of the Eight of Wands with you as you go.

ৰ EIGHT OF WANDS THEMES ৡ
sudden bursts of clarity, solutions to problems, clear communication, shining light on messy situations

EXERCISE
VISUALIZE SPEAKING YOUR TRUTH

Imagine a bright light radiating from your heart up through your throat whenever you speak—to what you are leaving behind, to yourself, and even to others about the situation you're leaving behind. Know that you are speaking from a bright, protected place of truth, even if your hands shake. The peace that comes after resolution is possible and it is near, and your courage will be rewarded with it.

EIGHT OF PENTACLES

Sweet relief! And don't you deserve it! Month 8 has been a doozy, right? If you were on the journey that the three previous Eights were taking you on, then this card represents the hard-earned peace that comes after the bravery of letting go.

Being a person who is gestating another person provides you with a direct ability to tap into what it is like to be incubated, held, unendingly nourished, and surrounded by the warmth of love.

Visualize how you are giving that to your baby, at all times, whether you're trying or not. Visualize how your body is nourishing and caring for your baby, how the warmth of your blood and love is surrounding them with potent, protective magic. Then transfer that visualization of loving warmth to yourself.

If it's possible, sit in a sunny spot where you can feel the warmth of the sun on your skin, or if that is unavailable to you at the moment, curl up in your favorite warm blanket. Allow yourself to feel surrounded. Recognize that you, too, are being incubated, soon to be rebirthed as a whole new person, as a parent (even if this isn't your first pregnancy, rebirth happens at all major life transitions). The gifts of our mother (the Earth) are here to be your nourishment—soak them up, ingest them.

Visualize the baby in your womb, and then visualize yourself in the world's womb. And know that you are just as protected, you are just as held, you are just as safe, and you are just as loved.

⊰ EIGHT OF PENTACLES THEMES ⊱

coming to a resolution, relief in what's been bothering you, feeling supported in your journey by Mother Earth, being rewarded for doing a hard thing, peace

TAROT SPREAD FOR LETTING GO

Pick out each of the Eights and lay them out in the following order: cups, swords, wands, pentacles.

Then pull a card to correspond with each Eight:

Under the Eight of Cups, ask: What it is that needs to be released?

Under the Eight of Swords, ask: What can I tend to in my soul to mitigate the fear of letting go?

Under the Eight of Wands, ask: How can I shed light and clarity on what feels complicated or fuzzy?

Under the Eight of Pentacles, ask: How can I come to a resolution on this?

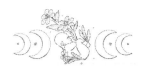

THE NINES

❧ MONTH 9 THEMES ❧

almost there; feeling pride in how far you've come physically, spiritually, emotionally; being wiser for what you've been through; manifestations coming to fruition; making the unconscious conscious; reflecting on the journey thus far; physical and emotional strength, instinctual decision-making

IN THE PHYSICAL BODY

This is the point in your pregnancy where your care provider is going to want your baby to be head down. Medicalized care providers may not recommend a physiologic birth if your baby is breech (not head down) because they frequently don't have the experience or much training in what to do in the event of a breech birth, other than to surgically remove the baby via surgical birth. Breech delivery is a lost (colonized) art that does have special requirements but is possible under the care of a knowledgeable care provider. A breech presentation is a variation of normal that a few practitioners still know how to handle, and perhaps you will need to seek a new care provider who is skilled in attending breech births.

If your baby is breech and a breech-competent provider is inaccessible to you, revisit the exercises covered in Month 4 (page 58), visit the Spinning Babies website (www.spinningbabies.com) for more techniques on turning your baby, continue chiropractic care (this has been helping with optimal positioning all along), and visit a prenatal acupuncturist.

This is a great time to remind you that your birth is your show. You are the sovereign of that space, and your care providers work *for* you. You can always say no. You can always wait and see. You still have options, even when things are presented in a way that makes you feel as if you have none.

NINE OF CUPS

You have squeezed every drop of juice to be squeezed out of the experience of this emotional journey. You rode every wave, honored every feeling, allowed yourself to cry every tear. You will never relate to your emotions the same way again now having experienced this powerful transformation, after having honestly seen it through, all the way to the end. Soon your body will do the work of unwrapping your prize at the end of this journey, but for now, pause and celebrate. Actively honor how far you've come on this particular trip, on this particular pregnancy.

It is likely that magic feels more present and available to you now for having gone through this journey than at the start. You did that. You harnessed that and pulled it into yourself. I'm proud of you!

You put in work and built emotional wealth. You did the brave, hard thing of shedding what did not serve you and what was not aligned with what your intuition knows to be right for you. The Nine of Cups then shows up as the reward for doing the brave and hard thing.

This card is a signal to pause and be proud of that work, but it also is a free pass to treat yourself. Of all the emotional, watery cups cards, this one feels the most grounded in the body to me. You'll get to be with your pregnant body only so much longer, and this card is indicative of bodily self-care in all the most clichéd ways we tend to think about self-care: give yourself permission to indulge in bubble baths or spiritual baths, prenatal massage, orgasms, delicious nourishing foods, and your favorite ways to take care of the physical body that has carried you through this emotional journey thus far. Refer to the Empress chapter (page 175) if you need help knowing what I mean by this. If you can't give yourself that permission to utterly spoil yourself, this card is giving you that permission.

⊰ NINE OF CUPS THEMES ⊱

deep self-care, honoring how far you've come, celebrating yourself, rest, having gained some emotional intelligence as a result of this emotional journey

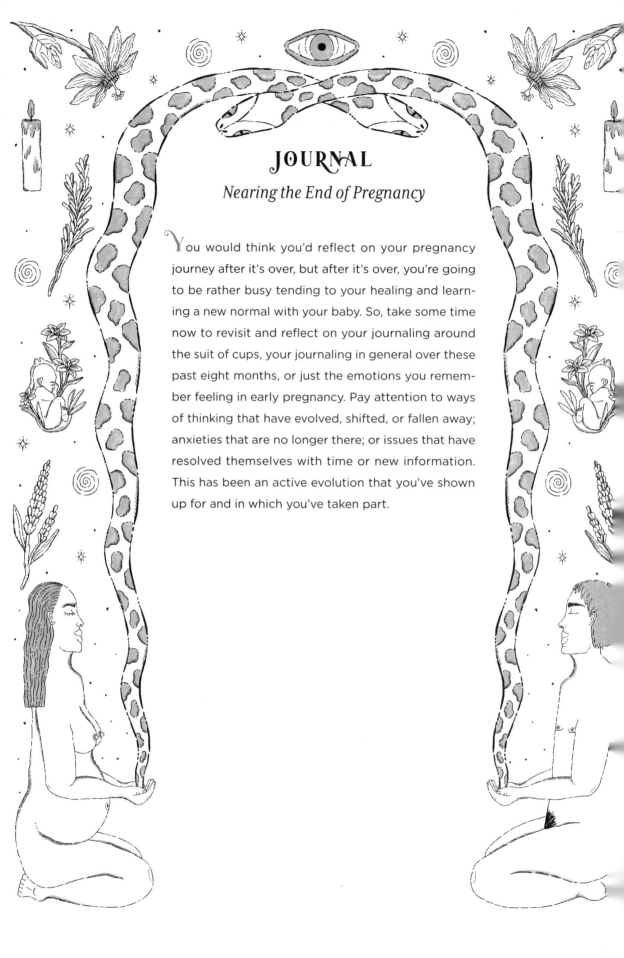

JOURNAL

Nearing the End of Pregnancy

You would think you'd reflect on your pregnancy journey after it's over, but after it's over, you're going to be rather busy tending to your healing and learning a new normal with your baby. So, take some time now to revisit and reflect on your journaling around the suit of cups, your journaling in general over these past eight months, or just the emotions you remember feeling in early pregnancy. Pay attention to ways of thinking that have evolved, shifted, or fallen away; anxieties that are no longer there; or issues that have resolved themselves with time or new information. This has been an active evolution that you've shown up for and in which you've taken part.

NINE OF WANDS

Our creativity is nearly at its peak, sparking a more primal way of being
and thinking (a primal instinct is showing up because we'll
need it to shine during labor). This could manifest as nesting, the instinct to create a space where you'll feel safe and
provided for postpartum. This could show up as an increase
in sexual desire, because your baby is ready to be born
soon, and your body is in fact ready to soon birth. The
contractions induced by orgasm can be a catalyst,
initiating cervical dilation. If you're having sex with
a partner who produces semen, the prostaglandins
in their semen work to soften the cervix, preparing the cervix to begin effacement (the thinning
of the cervix as it begins to expand). Inversely,
for the same reason, this instinct could show up as
lack of sexual desire, because your body knows
where your baby is in their development, more accurately
than any estimated due dates or sonograms, and maybe your
body wants to incubate your baby longer.

In a less clinical, but still scientific way, if you're feeling the desire
at all to tap into your sensuality right now, that is your instincts working on honing
that spirit-body connection and brushing up a major ally—your sexuality—that your
body has to cope with the intensity of labor. Wherever your instincts are steering
you, sex or no sex, nesting or no nesting, you can trust them.

The Nine of Wands cautions you against falling into the trap of "being just so *done*
with pregnancy." There is potent, powerful medicine in the waiting, in the liminal
space that is the final weeks of pregnancy. Being "over it," meaning over pregnancy
itself, can result in you conceding to unnecessary management of the onset of your
labor. Patience is the name of the game at this point; you worked too hard throughout this pregnancy to give in on any values-based choices you made about your desired birth.

Allow me to share some peony plant medicine with you that best articulates this
important card. Being a gardener and amateur herbalist, I observe so many similarities between the process of growing, budding, and blooming and the process of
pregnancy and birth. Peonies bring to mind two births I attended back-to-back as a

new doula. Both births had complications that caused labor to start early on its own. One of the births necessitated medical intervention, and one did not, unfolding on its own with patience and observation as a planned home birth. But in both cases, I was amazed at the body's ability to recognize that the baby was in duress, or would be in the near future, initiating labor before forty weeks.

It's no surprise that the same intuition exists across nature. I once bought a peony bush with a stem that was already budding but not yet in bloom. Unfortunately, the plant sustained an injury on the drive home from the greenhouse. As the care provider of this plant who has knowledge of what it takes for peonies to bloom, I assessed the damage, observing that enough of the stem was still intact to wait it out patiently, letting the bud mature enough to viably bloom. Sure enough, before any of the other buds on this bush bloomed, the damaged stem bloomed first. The plant recognized the damage and prioritized blooming the damaged bud early. The bloom was able to come full-term, having had the chance to open on its own.

My other option would have been to cut the stem when I noticed the damage, then do what's called "forcing" the bloom by sticking the stem in warm water in sunlight, and hoping it would open on its own. If it doesn't, you can peel back some of the outer green petals, working to encourage an early opening, but there is risk of further damage (in birth, this is the equivalent of inducing labor by performing a membrane sweep or manually dilating the cervix with a Foley balloon). Depending on how ready the bud is, forcing the bloom may or may not work. Why? Because peonies require that ants come in and eat the sticky coating off their tight, hard buds in order for the bud to be able to soften and open. This is how nature made peonies, producing the healthiest blooms when the process is able to naturally unfold. By leaving the stem on the bush, it got its fair share of ant activity, until the bush recognized that it was time for this bud to bloom early, and so it did.

In the cases of both births, the birthing people's bodies knew what to do by initiating labor early, and for one of the birthing people, it wasn't only her rapidly contracting uterus that knew what to do, but her intuition that guided her to go to the hospital sooner than she planned. And her intuition was correct because she did indeed have a placental abruption.[*]

....

[*] This is when the placenta begins to detach from the uterine wall before the baby has had a chance to be born. It is a rare condition, occurring in only about 1 percent of pregnant people. Sometimes there is no discernable cause for a placental abruption, but other times it is caused by a trauma or injury sustained while pregnant. The safest course of action during a placental abruption is swift surgical delivery.

With the other birthing person, the patience and observation of a knowledgeable care provider was what was needed, but ultimately, like my peony, she needed to be left alone to bloom on her own. Her baby was born with the veins from the umbilical cord spread out on the amniotic sac (a velamentous cord insertion).* This birthing person's body knew to initiate labor early because the bigger this baby got, the more strain would be put on those vital, unprotected veins. This birthing person's intuition had told her all throughout her pregnancy that this baby would be early, and her labor did indeed initiate just before thirty-eight weeks.

Nature unfolds the way it does for a reason, and there will always be some consequence—big or small—for interrupting it, trying to control it, thinking you know better than it. Sometimes that consequence is unavoidable. Sometimes careful risk-assessment analysis absolutely necessitates medical intervention. But whenever possible, patience, observation, and a deep knowledge of how nature intends for the process to unfold and why should inform the course of action (or more likely, inaction). Habit, protocol, profit, control, and schedules have no business informing the best course of action in birth or in blooming.

☌ NINE OF WANDS THEMES ⊱

when it comes to instincts, nothing is forced; potential increase in sexual interest; trusting your body; cautioning you against rushing to be done with pregnancy

NINE OF SWORDS

Fears and anxieties are being conjured by brain chemistry (again) but this time, it's as a sort of final hurrah. Your spirit knows it needs to detox these feelings *now* before they try to take the wheel of your labor and birth.

Let everything that comes up come up. Let it come in waves that rise and wash over you like the waves of your impending labor. I encourage you to share the fears that rise up, whenever they rise up, but just ensure that you're sharing your fears with someone who isn't going to project their own experiences on to you or panic and compromise your birth values and goals just because you shared your fears with them.

Don't get discouraged in a *Damn it, I thought I was over this fear!* kind of manner. In

---

* Normally, the two veins and an artery in the umbilical cord are all safely concentrated in that cord, connecting from the fetus and inserted in the center of the placenta. Concentrated in the cord, these veins are protected from damage or compression by the umbilical jelly (commonly known as Wharton's jelly) that surrounds them.

all likelihood, if you put in that previous work, you probably are past it. Spiraling back around to the same old fears is to be expected and you're getting a chance to flex your new skills. Now that you've done some healing, how are you going to handle these old fears? Probably not in the same way as you would in the past.

So, welcome the rising fears, don't shove them down. Your fear—that is, your brain—is only seeking to keep you safe, but in doing so, it's also going to try to keep you small. Approach your fears around labor and birth with understanding, gentleness, and maybe even gratitude. You can thank your fear for its concern, visualize wiping it away from wherever you feel your fear (often this will be your solar plexus, below your chest, but above your gut) and then visualize moving forward from your glowing, brave, beating heart instead.

Do not make decisions from a Nine of Swords place. There is always time for a pause—five minutes, an hour, a day, a week, whatever is needed to satisfy and settle how loud the voice of fear can feel.

ᛝ NINE OF SWORDS THEMES ᚠ
a final reprise of our fears and doubts, traumas coming to the surface to be cleared away, familiar problems, brain chemistry protecting you, detoxing from fear, taking your time to make big decisions

NINE OF PENTACLES

Much like the Nine of Cups, the Nine of Pentacles is asking you to pause and look at how far you've come on this journey of growth, this time in the literal sense.

Reflect on this journey within your physical body. Visually, remember when your pregnancy was an invisible notion that only you knew. A seed you'd planted, but all you could visibly see, water, or tend to was the dirt. Now just look how you've grown and bloomed. Just look at how you've alchemized nourishing food, water, oxygen, and your body's innate creative capabilities into the squirming little person beneath the surface of your skin. Go you!

Even though you're not at the fully bloomed completion that will be the Ten, this, too, is an accomplishment. Pause and honor it as such. I'm sure as hell celebrating you! Celebrate by treating yourself, or nourish your own energy with generosity to others. Give to others in a way that makes you feel good or give yourself permission to have an entire day devoted only to caring for your mind, body, and spirit.

If you're planning to birth at home, this is a lovely energy to invoke to curate a birth space that gives you a satisfied smile when you walk into it (playing into the possible nesting instinct of the Nine of Wands). If you're planning an out-of-home birth,* this is a lovely energy to invoke when packing your bag, including all the creature comforts that are uniquely necessary for you, even if it doesn't make sense to anyone else.

☽ NINE OF PENTACLES THEMES ☾
doing whatever makes you comfortable, recognizing your accomplishment,
in full bloom, making your environment cozy

SUGGESTED PACKING LIST FOR
AN OUT-OF-HOME BIRTH BAG

- a pretty robe, if pretty robes are your thing
- your comfiest, most stretchy bras
- lavender, clary sage, geranium, lemon, orange, vetiver essential oils (and a carrier oil for them)
- travel diffuser, if you don't plan on topically applying the essential oils
- your crystals, both those that look pretty to you and those that are shaped in a way that would be good for massaging pressure points during labor
- a houseplant or two that makes you smile every time you look at it (yes, I'm serious!)
- birth affirmation cards/visuals
- your favorite cozy blanket from home
- bone broths, birthing teas
- a speaker for music with your playlist already prepared (I recommend the melodious affirmation chanting of Beautiful Chorus)

----

* I like to use the term *out-of-home birth* because it's more historically factual. We typically call a hospital birth just "birth"—assuming that's where it will take place, and then if it takes place at home or a birth center, we call it an "out-of-hospital birth." In this way, we subconsciously (and consciously) position hospital birth as the norm, and anywhere else we might birth as the abnormal option, in need of a more specific alternative name. But birth began in the home and then was taken out of the home during the time of the Industrial Revolution and the colonization of midwifery (see the "History of Birth" chapter, page 125). Birthing in hospitals is a trend we've been doing for less than one hundred years. So, in the full spectrum of things, saying "out-of-home" birth for a hospital birth or birth center birth is more accurate.

- the obvious stuff: the baby clothes/blankets that you like best, the car seat already in the car, phone charger, deodorant (yours and your partner's), contact lens solution (yours and your partner's), toothbrush and paste (yours and your partner's), camera (if you're not having a birth photographer or just using your phone)

If it sounds like I'm suggesting that you make your labor and delivery room look like your own living room, then you're right, that's precisely what I'm suggesting. And it's not just so you look cute or so your birth photos look pretty. Labor and birth are a combination of mental and physical Olympics requiring a very specific mental state in addition to physical endurance. If you are dressed in a patient's robe, and only looking at a hospital room with all its sterility and beeping machinery, you're going to feel more like a hospital patient than a healthy birthing person. Because of the hormonal requirements for physiological birth, how you *feel* deeply affects how your experience will go. It is not selfish or superfluous. You are not a "diva" for planning for or requiring a curated, intentional space during birth. We need the comforting, pain-relieving hormone of oxytocin flowing freely and abundantly, not just for pain relief, but to keep labor moving along as expediently as possible. At all costs, we need to avoid introducing adrenaline, which will halt the flow of oxytocin and therefore increase pain or halt the progression of labor. Comfortable and feeling safe is the safest way for you to birth.

Here are some things you can't pack but should plan for in your birthing space: laughter, dancing, slow walks, deep long hugs, hair strokes, and anything else that makes you feel like a whole human who is loved.

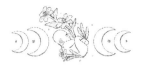

THE TENS

"A comprehensive postpartum plan is NOT:
- Your partner getting 2 to 4 days off work (if you're lucky).
- Your mom who lives down the road, visiting you once or twice.
- Relatives from all over the place popping in to hold the baby.

A comprehensive postpartum plan IS:
- Knowing how birth impacts your body, mind, and emotions.
- Setting your own expectations and boundaries.
- Having daily help in place to support your healing.
- Warm, nourishing meals that are easy to access.
- Gathering your resources for healing ahead of time."

—Raeanne Madison, MPH, Bois Forte Band of Chippewa Indians,
Postpartum Healing Lodge

⊰ MONTH 10 THEMES ⊱

completion, stepping into a new self and a new way of being, writing a new story about ourselves from scratch, no going back, navigating a new brain chemistry and internal landscape, possibility of spiraling negativity when fear is introduced, radiant joyful love, fulfillment of the journey started in the Aces, blooming of the flower from the seeds planted in the Aces, opening of the gift given in the Aces, your story going from hypothetical and hoped for to being written, isolation, taking on too much and learning how to manage our loads, a family is born, what we've learned will live on, full circle, a return to the Fool for both yourself and your baby, birth from your baby's perspective and how to ease the transition for them

IN THE PHYSICAL BODY

All these past months the growth of your baby and your belly was slow and steady, and then *bam!* Here comes labor, birth, the start of postpartum, bodyfeeding (if that applies to you), and everything else you've been anticipating.

Physically, oxytocin will be flowing through your body during labor, helping things progress, doing its part to mitigate the intense sensations, and then eventually assisting in bonding and the start of bodyfeeding. Prostaglandins are present during labor to soften the cervix and aid in effacement (as I mentioned, prostaglandins are found naturally in semen), as are endorphins, which can transmute the intense sensation of perceived pain into the possibility of pleasure. The pineal gland naturally produces dimethyltryptamine (DMT) during three intensely vulnerable experiences where we are being called to surrender: during orgasm, while giving birth, and during death.

Production of cortisol (the stress hormone) during labor does not support the other necessary hormones that keep labor progressing and reduce the perception of pain. In an out-of-home birth setting, beeping machines and disruptive monitoring can instill fear in the birthing parent about the safety of their baby, which can result in cortisol or adrenaline production. Frequent visits and proddings from nurses can feel irritating and cause the production of cortisol. I've heard nurses joke that they "scared the contractions away" when they are unable to get their routine read of fetal heart tones during a contraction. It's not funny because it's true–the mere presence of strangers can halt contractions.

Additionally, the production of adrenaline during labor is oxytocin's nemesis. Doula and educator Latham Thomas calls fear and anxiety birth's "kryptonite." Biologically, if your body is producing adrenaline because of fear, your body is going to assume there must be a threat or danger that you need to escape, so it will halt labor so you can inhabit adrenaline's "flight or fight" mode and get yourself somewhere safe. As adrenaline assists you in running away or fighting, it sends all your blood rushing to your outer extremities and away from your internal organs, which your baby is currently inhabiting. Introducing fear into your birth setting can even cause your baby to be in distress for this reason.

All these helpful and unhelpful hormones during labor and birth are why it's not just a nice idea for your birthing space to be comfortable and as safe feeling as possible to you (recognizing that what feels "safe" might not be the same for every birthing body), for your entire birth team (including any family members present) to be supportive and knowledgeable about the requirements of physiologic birth, and for the birthing position, setting, tone, and so on to be led by the person doing the actual birthing. These things are necessary for promoting an optimally safe birth, not superfluous luxuries. You have a right to require that the needs of your physical body are met during birth and postpartum.

If you are able to and planning to feed your baby from your own breasts or chest, then the hormones prolactin and oxytocin are needed for that physiologic function to occur. Again, stress (and the cortisol it produces) can interfere with or even halt the production of these hormones, and therefore halt the process of lactation. Fears about whether your baby is getting enough—your newborn's stomach is the size of a marble and colostrum is dense and highly nutritious for them—can actually stall your body's ability to make the more liquid-like, hydrating milk that comes in two to four days postpartum. It's not unusual for this more obvious milk to not come in until you're at home again and in your own comfortable space.

TEN OF CUPS

A new family is born. Even if this isn't your first baby, this family, in this iteration, never existed before, now that this new human or new story has been introduced to the world.

You went on this emotional journey that the Ace of Cups presented you, so it might seem paradoxical that you are now in a space of feeling such unmitigated emotions so freely. But this was never meant to be a journey to learn how to control your emotions. This was a journey to learn how to allow your emotional self to be fully integrated into who you are. This was a journey to set your emotions free.

This card, like the full moon, will be what you can tap into to harness a greater power for birthing than you even knew you had in you. Then it is the big, surging emotional release of birth, the apex of the pregnancy journey. *Anyone else ever cry when they have an orgasm sometimes? No? Just me?*

And then the energy of this card stays with us as our gentle ally in postpartum when we are having some capital-*F* Feelings. There are likely a lot of tears that you can't name as either "happy" tears or "sad" tears, and it's because they are truly neither and both. This point in the cups' journey speaks to an intensity of feeling that is so overwhelming we don't have words for it. It is enormous love, relief, satisfaction, and fulfillment all mixed with a melancholy mourning of the pregnancy experience and who we were before this experience (and possibly the loss of a desired birth story, or any other change of plans that can be cause for heartache).

I liken Ten of Cups to graduation—no matter how ready you were to be done with school, you likely still felt a tinge of melancholy over saying goodbye to your friends and teachers. Closing a chapter, or ending a book, is both satisfying, fulfilling, and a little sad, too, and that's okay. Let all the feelings flow. You're not obligated to name them; you're only asked to let them be expressed to the fullest.

In postpartum, the Ten of Cups is a reminder to care for ourselves with the same loving kindness that we do our newborn. When your baby was born, you were reborn too. A new version of yourself is calling for you to slowly step into a new normal. In addition to learning how to parent the new additional human in your home, remember to parent yourself.

Prioritize feeding yourself at whatever frequency your body calls for, drink plenty of water, because we feed our babies as often as they ask, right? Be just as attentive to your own needs. When we are parenting ourselves, we are allowing any emotions that arise to speak their peace and flow through us. We don't yell at our babies to stop crying just because we don't understand the source of the tears, right? When you are parenting yourself, you are asking for all the hugs, community, and sensitive support you need. We would never tell our brand-new babies that they don't deserve to be held and comforted through big transitions or emotions.

Everything you need to know about how to properly parent yourself is likely already in the actions you're taking to tenderly care for your newborn, acclimating them from a watery womb to being a breathing, dry-land human. Transitions are always hard, and this learning curve is particularly steep for both of you.

There is no pressure. Go at your own pace, listen to your baby and your body, and give both what they need. Frustration is expected, but don't pressure or expect yourself to be somewhere you aren't right now. There will come a time for leaving the house. There will come a time for showing off your cute, chunky babe to the world. There will come a time for all the cute stuff you planned to do with your baby, but in the first several weeks after birth, if you're feeling like you're not ready for that just yet, honor it. You just did tremendous work growing a baby and birthing them, and you deserve the sweet reward of recuperation.

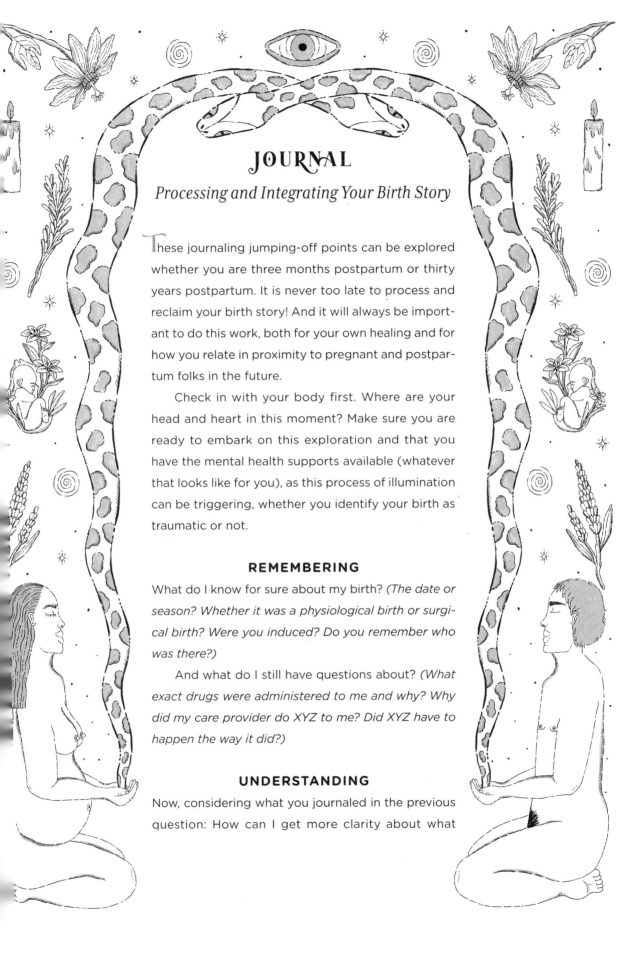

JOURNAL

Processing and Integrating Your Birth Story

These journaling jumping-off points can be explored whether you are three months postpartum or thirty years postpartum. It is never too late to process and reclaim your birth story! And it will always be important to do this work, both for your own healing and for how you relate in proximity to pregnant and postpartum folks in the future.

Check in with your body first. Where are your head and heart in this moment? Make sure you are ready to embark on this exploration and that you have the mental health supports available (whatever that looks like for you), as this process of illumination can be triggering, whether you identify your birth as traumatic or not.

REMEMBERING

What do I know for sure about my birth? *(The date or season? Whether it was a physiological birth or surgical birth? Were you induced? Do you remember who was there?)*

And what do I still have questions about? *(What exact drugs were administered to me and why? Why did my care provider do XYZ to me? Did XYZ have to happen the way it did?)*

UNDERSTANDING

Now, considering what you journaled in the previous question: How can I get more clarity about what happened during my birth that I still don't fully understand? *(Can I research the evidence around a medication or procedure that was used? Can I ask someone who was present? Can I ask for my birth chart/medical records from my care provider? Can I consult a trusted birth professional who has a deep understanding of birth to gain a new perspective?)*

What new understanding have I gained through my digging and research? *(Was something I experienced necessary or unnecessary? Was something I experienced "standard practice" but not evidence-based? Did I experience medical racism? Have I found anyone else who has had a similar experience to mine?)*

INTEGRATING

What (if anything) about my child's personality is reflected in their birth story?

How can I integrate that information into how I parent my child?

How has my birth story impacted (or not impacted) how I show up as a parent?

RECLAIMING

What is different about me now as opposed to who I was before I went through the birth portal? *(You might feel the urge to view some of these things as "good," for example: "I found my voice and learned how to set boundaries"; or you might view some of them as "bad," for example: "I'm paranoid about medical care providers now and I don't trust them with my child's care." But try not to assign a "good" or "bad" designation to who you are now after your birth experience. The results or who you are now after birth are neutral. There are ways you have coped and survived what you went through, no matter how you view your birth story.)*

What does my birth story teach me about how I am meant to show up in the world to fulfill my soul's purpose (if at all)?

Note: While I think nearly everyone's healing journey can benefit from remembering, understanding, and integrating, not everyone can or will want to take it to the final step of reclaiming. Especially if there were experiences of trauma involved in your birth story, it's not always recommended to "transcend" the trauma or look for the lesson in it. Depending on the situation, this can easily slip into spiritual bypassing* that can result in gaslighting† your own self into thinking that your trauma "needed to happen that way" for you to learn the lesson, be who you are now, learn your purpose, and so on. I do not condone that kind of thinking, and it's why I suggest that this work should potentially be undergone with the support and guidance of a mental health professional, if that makes sense for you.

In short, if reclamation makes sense for you, by all means. But if reclamation doesn't make sense for you, if a shitty birth experience is just that and nothing more, you are no less healed, no less enlightened than the next person who chose to make meaning. We all have different means of coping with our experiences, and we all deserve to be validated, however that looks for each of us as individuals.

----

* See "Glossary of Terms," page xvii, for the definition of *spiritual bypassing*.

† "Gaslighting" refers to a manipulation tactic to make you question your own reality.

TEN OF WANDS

Only you can do the work of opening your bodily vessel to be a conduit for a new human to come through—but it's not a load you have to carry alone. Lean on your people. Lean into your team. Don't lift a finger for a single thing that is not required of you personally.

Move your body however you need to, and if you're in an out-of-home birth setting, on a continuous fetal monitor that needs to be adjusted every time you move, then move however you want or need to anyway, and let the nurses come adjust it as needed. And don't apologize when they have to come in for the ump-teenth time. If your doula is getting tired of doing hip squeezes, have them switch off with your partner, while they refresh your cold washcloth, hug you, and stroke your hair. If it's not already flowing freely, you can ask for the verbal encouragement you need to keep going. And I'm not talking about the whole room yelling "Push!" at you. I'm talking about affirmations like *That was a good contraction, that one did a lot of work, keep going, you're doing beautifully. I'm in awe of the strength and power you're harnessing right now. You're going to be such a good parent, I can't wait to see it.*

There might be a point in labor where it is too much, where it's too heavy, where it overwhelms you. Know that it is supposed to be this way, and even in this other-worldly enormity, you are safe. Give your fears and doubts away to someone you know won't compromise on your values after hearing them. If there's no one in the room to whom you can cry *I can't do it anymore* without them rushing to give you pain relief, or if you're already using pain medication but are just so exhausted and over it that you're feeling ready to opt for unwanted surgical birth, or even if you're being wheeled back for surgical birth and you're afraid, give up these fears to your ances-tors, your guides, your loved ones who are passed. Know they are there with you, holding you. You do not have to carry the weight of your fears or the intensity alone, even if it feels like no one physically present can hear you or see your intensity with-out looking away.

⊰ TEN OF WANDS THEMES ⊱

feeling the enormous intensity of labor, feeling like giving up, being divinely supported, asking for help in labor, birth support

A LITTLE NOTE FOR BIRTH PARTNERS AND DOULAS

In my experience, I've found one of the most underrated comfort tools is eye contact, which is why our presence (actually *there* and *with* them, not constantly looking at our phones or machinery) is so important.

When a person in the throes of labor looks into your eyes during the peak of their surge's intensity, don't look away. You need to be steady and grounding for them. We are culturally so uncomfortable with this kind of power that we inherently want to shy away from it, to avert our gaze. But I implore you to stay.

I have had birthing folks bore into my very soul with their gaze during a surge, nearly bringing me to my knees and making me want to weep. But they are asking for you to be in the enormity of their intensity with them. And it is a gift for you to stay with them in it. They are the only ones who can do the work of birth, but seeing and acknowledging the work they are doing by remaining present with them is one way you can make them feel safe and lessen their load.

Suggested Birth Affirmations for Birthing Partners to Say

- "You are safe."
- "Thank you for working so hard to bring this new soul into our community/ family."
- "You are so strong, so much stronger than you ever knew before."
- When they say they can't do it: "You already are doing it."
- "This isn't forever. Look how far you've come already."
- "It's okay to cry if you need to."

Other Coping Measures for Birth Partners to Try During Labor

(See the Tower chapter, page 214, for more about the purpose of pain and for an expanded version of coping techniques.)

- Hot or cold washcloths on their forehead, chest, or lower back (check in with the birthing person about what temperature is preferred for them at that moment). Always apply cold/hot compresses with a strong assured hand pressing down to ground them. Bonus: Apply a little lavender or clary sage essential oil to the wet washcloth for aromatherapeutic effects as well.

- Holding their hand. Much like eye gazing, this is an underrated form of supporting birthing people, and is a way to signify that you are there with them.

- Hip squeezes or a fist applied to the middle of their lower back. Always check in with the birthing person about what is feeling good for them. Placing your open palms on either side of the birthing person's hips during a contraction can help open their pelvic bones, provide relief, and relieve back labor. Counterpressure in the tailbone can provide relief at a certain point as well. As long as you've obtained consent from the birthing person, do not be afraid to touch them with a strong and reassuring hand.

- Eyebrow massage. It is helpful for cervical dilation for birthing people to have relaxed facial features and a relaxed jaw. If their brow is furrowed or jaw is tight, massaging their brow and jaw between contractions can help them remember to relax and soften. The same is true for a shoulder massage.

- Acupressure points. Do some research prior to labor about what acupressure points can be massaged to relieve pain during labor.

- Offer them something to eat. Many hospitals are still carrying the archaic policy* of no food and drink during labor, despite the evidence that shows this practice to be outdated and even unsafe. Birth is a highly athletic event, and it's normal to need food that actually gives you energy, not just ice chips and juice. Honey sticks, bone broth, fruit, coconut water or anything that sounds good to the birthing person should be offered at regular intervals to help keep up their strength.

....

* The "no food and drink" policy is a relic from the "Twilight Sleep" era where birthing people were knocked out completely, thus they could potentially aspirate their own vomit while they were prostrate and alone on intense drugs that are no longer used. The concern now is that if an emergency Cesarean section were needed, vomit aspiration could potentially occur on a fully anesthetized birthing person. But the act of withholding food from birthing people in the first place can create an emergency. Being nourished to have enough energy and endurance during labor is emergency prevention. And there's even recent evidence to show that being under anesthesia on an empty stomach carries just as much risk of vomit aspiration. So, as always, research the evidence prior to birth, and make sure to indicate it on your birth plan whether you would like to eat or not eat during labor.

TEN OF SWORDS

While it could of course be applied to labor and birth, too, this card resonates most for me during postpartum time. Because this card speaks to painful endings, loss, and even betrayal.

It is not typically a part of the evolved, modern interpretation of the Ten of Swords to still include the notion of betrayal, but it is not unlikely that at some point during your immediate postpartum period, you will utter the words, "Nobody told me . . ." and then fill in the blank with any number of things: *Nobody told me I might experience cracked nipples. Nobody told me about the anxiety about whether my newborn poops enough. Nobody told me that interrupted sleep would become my new normal for a while and that it doesn't mean anything is wrong with my baby. Nobody told me about "brick dust" and that it looks like there's blood in my newborn's diaper!* I could go on and on.

And in this way, part of the postpartum experience can feel like its own kind of betrayal. Why the hell did people gift us so many silly baby gadgets instead of just being here to spoon-feed me soup while I nourish a human from my body endlessly? Where are the people who were so excited for me to be pregnant now, in the wreckage that can be learning a new normal with a new human and fresh bodily wounds and depleted nutrients?

And as for loss and painful endings, some of us might experience a more tangible, tragic loss, like the loss of a desired birth plan or even the loss of a child. But it is my belief that the kind of loss that the Ten of Swords is indicating is the loss of a previous self,* which will almost certainly befall you after the birth of your child. Attempting to fit ourselves back into that shell that we outgrew is part of what is causing the pain, struggle, and strife.

We might want to "get our body back" or "get our life back," but guess what? *This* body is still *your* body, and *this* life is still *your* life. You're living it, you're doing it. I'm going to go ahead and boldly say that the idea that you could ever be the same after the life-shaking experiences of creating a human and birthing it, then figuring out how to raise that human, is pretty ridiculous and impossible. Of course we will be moved and utterly changed by this journey. Of course we will lose who we were before we were so moved by these experiences. Something new is growing in place of that previous self but it is still nascent at this point.

....

* A trusted soul tarot reader and teacher, Lindsey Mack, says on their podcast *Tarot for the Wild Soul*, in the episode about the Ten of Swords (an episode that has helped evolve and enrich my interpretation of this card), that there is no going back to the previous self that is being left behind in the Ten of Swords.

I don't say all that to bypass or diminish the difficulty of the energy in this card. It's likely that only time and gentleness with yourself will ease the discomfort of inhabiting a new person that doesn't feel like you. Until eventually it feels like a more authentic you than you ever even knew, not necessarily because of parenthood, but because of the enormity of this transformation you just went through.

☽ TEN OF SWORDS THEMES ☾

loss of previous self, despair, difficult adjustments, steep learning curve,
feeling betrayed, acceptance of the new self as a parent

HERBAL SITZ BATH TEA

Like the other recipes for herbal infusions, you do not necessarily need to have every ingredient on this list in order to make a healing sitz bath tea. And likewise, if you do a simple Google search there are more herbs than these that you can use if you prefer!

INGREDIENTS

1 Tbsp comfrey (Traditionally to aid in wound healing, particularly in protecting against the incorrect development of scar tissue. This herb can be used as "herbal stitches" for minor tears and lacerations that occur during vaginal birth, but use caution on very deep wounds, as the external application can cause the outside of the tissue to heal first before the wound has healed deeper internally.)

1 Tbsp witch hazel (A natural astringent, this herb is soothing and anti-inflammatory, which can reduce swelling while healing, treat hemorrhoids, and provide comfort to the vulva when used as a compress.)

1 Tbsp yarrow (Known to stop bleeding in wounds and treat hemorrhoids. It also decreases risk of infection.)

1 Tbsp horsetail (Horsetail can be used both topically and internally [see Nutritious Herbal Infusion for Postpartum Healing, page 120] to help promote healing, particularly if you experienced perineal or vulval tears during birth, or a Cesarean birth. Horsetail is high in silica, which

is helpful in the production and repair of connective tissues, which can
accelerate healing.)

1 Tbsp plantain leaf (See Soothing Belly Rub, page 86, for how to gather
plantain leaf and more ways to prepare them. I have used plantain
leaf, my favorite herb as a parent, for everything from cracked
and blistered nipples to minor burns, cuts and
scrapes, diaper rash, bug bites, and eczema.
During postpartum, this herb shines in
helping soothe and heal tears, discomfort,
and inflammation after birth. It is naturally
antiseptic, which helps prevent infection
at the site of the tear. As a bonus, plantain
commonly grows wild in the Northern
Hemisphere, which makes accessing your own
for free relatively easy, depending on where you
live. It is not endangered and is often treated like a
weed by folks who don't know how useful it is.)

1 Tbsp calendula (Calendula flowers are antifungal, antibacterial,
antiseptic, and anti-inflammatory, which makes them perfect to aid
in healing the perineum after birth while reducing the risk of infection.
Calendula flowers can be made into a salve and used for sore nipples and
diaper rash too!)

1 Tbsp lavender (Not only does it smell amazing and have a calming effect
on the nervous system, it can also help heal irritated skin with its anti-
inflammatory and antiseptic properties.)

1 Tbsp rose petals (Rose petals smell amazing and will be soothing every
time you use your sitz bath tea, but they are also astringent, which can help
tonify the skin.)

1 Tbsp sea salt (Natural sea salt is healing and cleansing. You can also use
Epsom salts, just make sure it's not the kind that has any fragrance or oils
in it.)

DIRECTIONS

Add the ingredients to a large pot of boiling water, and then turn off the heat, cover with a lid, and allow to steep for a few hours.

After it has steeped long enough and the temperature of the liquid is warm but no longer hot, strain the liquid through a cheesecloth or fine-mesh strainer. Use some warm right away, and then store the rest in the refrigerator for later use.

THERE ARE SEVERAL WAYS TO USE YOUR SITZ BATH TEA NOW:

1. You can put this warm liquid directly into your peri-bottle (this is a special squirt bottle that will come in your birth kit if you're having a home birth, or you will get sent home from the hospital with one). After every time you urinate, spray this warm liquid directly onto your vulva instead of wiping with dry toilet paper (you can also spray while you are urinating to prevent the burning sensation that comes with urinating after vaginal birth).

2. You can spray this tea mixture into your pads to keep that healing compress held against your vulva and perineum. Some folks will freeze pads with this mixture on them because cold does feel nice when you have a painful and inflamed perineum, but ultimately, cold does not promote blood flow and therefore does not promote healing, so it is recommended to use the sitz bath tea when it is warm.

3. You can do an actual sitz bath. This is a plastic bowl with a large rim that fits over your toilet and allows you to sit in a shallow bath of your sitz tea. Each sitz bath will come with instructions about how to use yours specifically.

4. Or you can take a makeshift sitz bath in your own bathtub (as long as it is clean and sanitary). Fill up your tub with a couple of inches of warm water, pour in your sitz bath tea while it is still warm, and sit in the healing herbs for 20 to 30 minutes.

TEN OF PENTACLES

In birth, and in parenthood, you are getting a glimpse into how the Earth feels about us, its children. Depending on your relationship with your parents, you're maybe even getting a glimpse into how your parents felt about you. This is one of those moments in life when things come full circle. This is an end that is also a beginning.

In staring into the wise eyes of your newborn, it becomes easier to tangibly imagine passing on your life's wisdoms to the new child, to see yourself as their elder one day. If you happened to birth a baby who has a uterus, their eggs were already developed inside them, while they were still inside you (and likewise, the egg that alchemized to make you not only existed inside your birth parent, but also existed inside your birth grandparent too), in an awesome, infinite, spiraling inception of life.

You might be breathless holding your baby in your arms and have no idea what to do next or where to go from here. You might still be living moment by precious moment. It can feel like you planned everything up until right now, so now what? But not having a plan at this point is okay. You just completed an enormous feat, no matter how your birth story unfolded. Allow your mind to merely meditate on what is. This is one way to really *live* into life and push the edges of what you thought was reality. You're doing it; you're living it. Well done.

NUTRITIOUS HERBAL INFUSION
FOR POSTPARTUM HEALING

Whether you have some or all of these ingredients, you can make your own customized herbal infusion or tea to support your healing postpartum and help fill in the gaps of nutrient depletion if you are bodyfeeding.

INGREDIENTS

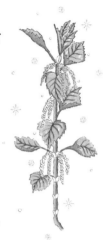

1 Tbsp nettles (For the same reason nettles are helpful during pregnancy, they are still helpful postpartum, namely for the boost in iron. In a vaginal birth, 250 to 500 ccs of blood loss is normal, and during a Cesarean surgical birth, up to 1,000 ccs of blood loss is normal. So, we need to build back up that blood postpartum, no matter how your birth went! Nettles will support your milk as well if you choose to bodyfeed, as it contains vitamin K, the necessary nutrient naturally found in our bodies that allows blood to clot, which babies don't produce in significant amounts until they're eight days old.)

1 Tbsp oatstraw (A nervine that supports the nervous system and eases stress through the big transition from pregnancy to parenthood. The calcium in oatstraw can enrich your milk if you're bodyfeeding as well. The other vitamins and minerals in oatstraw help replenish nutrients and promote restful sleep postpartum.)

1 Tbsp alfalfa (This herb has many nutrients, can curb nausea, can increase milk production, and can even limit excessive bleeding.)

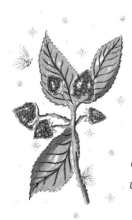

1 Tbsp red raspberry leaf (Tones the uterus, and therefore during the postpartum period can assist in the uterus's work to contract back down to prepregnancy size and minimize bleeding. The vitamins and minerals present in red raspberry leaf will also be helpful in replenishing nutrients lost during pregnancy and birth, and the vitamin B_6 found in this herb helps with mood intensity and irritability. Red raspberry leaf may be contraindicated if you have polycystic ovary syndrome [PCOS], uterine fibroids, or endometriosis.)

1 Tbsp red dates (Used in traditional Chinese medicine for general womb health but in particular during the postpartum lying-in period because of their womb-warming benefits, red dates are also highly nutritious, containing significant amounts of vitamins C, A, B₁, and B₂, protein, magnesium, calcium, iron, and phosphorus. Red dates enrich and replenish the blood to help support the body in restoring nutrients lost during pregnancy and birth and to support bodyfeeding. You can steep these and drink them as a tea by themselves or steep them in your bone broth recipes or herbal infusions. I prefer to cut or tear them in half and remove the seed to allow for maximum absorption into the infusion.)

1 Tbsp goji berries (We can give credit again to traditional Chinese medicine for knowing the benefits of goji berries during postpartum. Goji berries are powerful antioxidants that are helpful in protecting your immunity. They increase blood circulation [and therefore may be contraindicated if you are on blood thinners], nourish the kidneys and liver, stabilize blood sugar, and elevate moods. They can be eaten on yogurt or in oatmeal, you can drink them as a tea or add them into your herbal infusions.)

1 Tbsp hibiscus (Hibiscus is a galactagogue, meaning a substance that supports and promotes lactation. It treats high blood pressure, and so it can help protect against postpartum hypertension and is therefore not indicated if you have low blood pressure. Energetically and medicinally, hibiscus tends to the heart, which I find to be helpful in supporting and soothing the intensity of moods postpartum.)

1 Tbsp horsetail (Horsetail can be used both topically and internally to promote healing, particularly if you experienced perineal or vulval tears during birth, or a Cesarean birth. Horsetail is high in silica, which is helpful in the production and repair of connective tissues, which can accelerate healing.)

or 1 handful premade mixture of some or all these herbs

Raw honey or blackstrap molasses for sweetening

EQUIPMENT

Large stainless steel or glass pot
Cheesecloth or fine-mesh strainer
Glass jar with lid
Funnel

DIRECTIONS

To make an infusion: Bring a large stainless steel or glass pot of water to a boil, add your herbs, stir, turn off the heat, cover, and then allow to steep. For an infusion, you can steep anywhere from 4 to 12 hours. The longer it steeps, the more nutrients will be extracted from the herbs.

When you're ready to strain, place a funnel lined with cheesecloth or a strainer in a glass jar and strain the liquid into the jar. Try to squeeze as much liquid out of the herbs in the cloth or strainer as possible, as those last few drops out of the herbs are highly potent medicine!

Then, you can sweeten to taste with raw honey or blackstrap molasses (which is also high in iron). If you still find the tea not to your taste for regular drinking, you can cut it with juice or lemonade. Store it in the refrigerator for up to a week. Ask your postpartum support team to keep a batch of this brewed up regularly so that way you can have at least one glass a day.

To make tea: While an infusion is nice for maximum nutrient extraction from the extended steeping time, tea is nice because you can drink it hot and you don't need to store it. You can use 1 Tbsp herb mixture to 1 cup hot water, allow it to steep for 10 to 15 minutes, strain, sweeten with raw honey if you prefer, and then drink while warm. Warm food and beverages during the postpartum period are ideal to promote blood flow, digestion, proper healing, and bringing warmth back to the body that is lost when you are no longer pregnant.

"I chose this work [birthwork] because I want Black and Indigenous people to remember who they are and the power they continue to hold by simply existing today . . . We can and will reclaim what is ours. Our bodies are ours. Our babies are ours. We must do the necessary work to reclaim, honor, and heal. For ourselves and for the next generations to come."

—Mariah Eldridge, Nizhóní Sol Birthwork

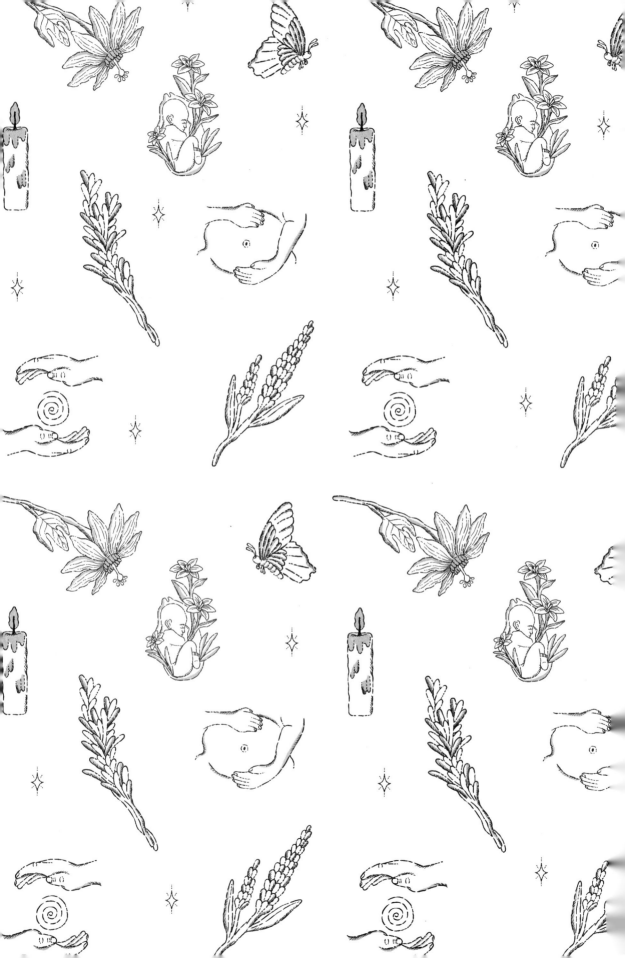

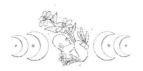

THE HISTORY OF BIRTH IN THE UNITED STATES

BY DR. STEPHANIE MITCHELL, "DOCTOR MIDWIFE"

A WORD ON TERMINOLOGY

Language shapes our experiences and has the potential to cause harm to others when used incorrectly or without thinking through the implications. In acknowledgment of the diversity among those who gestate and birth, I aim to use gender-inclusive language where possible. I recognize that the term maternal may omit childbearing people who do not identify as mothers from the narrative, from public health considerations, and from data, and we find ourselves in the midst of a system that continues to rely on this term in larger public and international health spheres. It is important for me to be cognizant and vigilant about both completely supporting folks who identify as women and mothers, and those childbearing persons who do not but find themselves suffering under the same failed health care systems as others.

We won't go back too far. We could, because people have been birthing babies since the dawn of time. Birth was depicted in ancient hieroglyphics, and midwifery was referred to in biblical manuscripts. Also, since the same dawn of time, the world has had an interesting relationship with how people enter this world through labor and birth. The nuances of pregnancy, labor, and birth are distinct and, at bare minimum, are based on one's precise location on the planet and place in time. Historically, most birth attendants have been women, but through the development of time and through recent modern-day obstetrics, we don't see that same relationship as much anymore.

Typical pregnancy care, labor, and birth that we experience today is inseparably linked to the history of midwifery. The United States in particular has a tangled, intricate, and sometimes painful history with how children are brought into this living, breathing realm and certainly with those who birthed these babies. From the first births that occurred in the then-wilderness of North America, where women inevitably were cared for by the resourceful Indigenous inhabitant midwives of the land or, when possible older, perhaps more experienced women who were knowledgeable as birth attendants. In the same token of variety, birth looked different for women who were birthing for the entirety of the period of the American Enslavement of kidnapped and human-trafficked Africans from the 1600s through to 1865 and then beyond. It was during this time that labors and births were most commonly attended by other enslaved women, often elder women, who came to have birth-attendant skills through personal experience or apprenticeship. With particular skill sets, some of these women were called midwives. These are just a few early American stories of labor and birth; there are many, as the backdrop of birth continued throughout the budding nation and birth was happening everywhere! In fact, each generation has stories of how typical labor and birth occurred as the norm. As a new generation is born, stories of how birth is accomplished will inevitably vary, sometimes starkly from the immediate generation before it. In the 1700s, it was thought that a man's right testicle and a woman's right ovary were responsible for making male children. See, things change. People learn, things improve, we obtain better understandings. That's how it's supposed to work.

By 1765 it was still mostly midwives, and some doctors, who delivered most babies, and it was almost always at birthing people's own homes. Around this same time the first formal training of midwives began, as hospital nurses received specialized obstetrical training. There was also a measurable growth of the American elite, which included American male doctors, and also some foreign-trained male doctors, who had come to America to practice. These influences had come to favor a more medical approach that accompanied a physician birth. Of note, just to give you an idea of where we are: It was also common and encouraged during the seventeenth and eighteenth centuries to sip on a brew of alcohol and oatmeal for restoration of energy after a particularly physically taxing labor. So, this is just a reminder that the recommendations and the norms change along the way. It wasn't until the 1800s that men were even invited into the birth space. And in those cases where they were present, they were advised not to look at the woman. A generation comes, and a generation goes. Things continue to change, advancements are made, and many things are learned and modified upon examination and study of best practice and a review of outcomes, successes, and failures. We do the best we can with what we have at the time for knowledge and resources.

In the 1900s, midwives delivered about half of the babies that were born. And still, barring nearly exceptional circumstances, 100 percent of babies born were at home. The largest shift occurred during the 1920s with an increase in requirements for licensure and regulations for midwives, the institution of medical schools, and subsequently, an increase in available physicians. So much so that only fifteen years later, in 1935, those with the means to pay for hospital services utilized physicians to deliver their babies in hospitals. This was largely due to the use of anesthesia, which had become popularized and improved as a method of pain control in labor, in conjunction with the loss of the American midwife from their respective communities. It became the poor working class, and those who were not invited to utilize "whites only" hospitals, that had their births attended to by midwives. In a forty-year span, the utilization of midwives dropped to about 15 percent of births by 1940.

When television was popularized in the 1950s and '60s, visual media representations commonly depicted birth as an event you didn't witness on screen. We might see men in the waiting rooms of a busy hospital ward smoking cigars. Perhaps a uniformed nurse or a white-coat-clad physician enters to pronounce congratulatory remarks to the room of either nervously pacing fathers (newbies) or jovial waiting men (not their first rodeo). "Mr. Smith, it's a boy!" they might exclaim. It was during the time of these popularized anesthetized births, where the mother was nonpresent in the process, or present as an afterthought. This was often referred to as "twilight birth." It was a common and desirable birth that was advertised as the dignified way to birth. Certain interventions such as heavy anesthesia, episiotomies, and mid- or high-pelvic forceps-assisted vaginal deliveries were normalized in order to accomplish the task of birth, regardless of the effect or outcomes it had on those who utilized these services. That was the part that was not advertised.

Like many other fields of medicine, obstetrics is a specialty practice. It has changed, and improved, and specialized, and nearly perfected some interventions, while improving outcomes of many situations that would have fared poorly without the resources and domain that is obstetrics and the maternal fetal medicine specialty. Many of the innovations have brought about great improvements, but we'd also be remiss not to mention that many of the advancements to improve this science are the same as most methods of improvement. They are made through trial and error. Trial and error means that someone, somewhere, was on the error side as a result of the medicalizing and industrialization of the labor and birth process. These advancements were made at the expense of bodies through which learning was not a consensual act. This is no different from many other fields of medicine in that regard, but in obstetrics, people of child-bearing age and their babies are the target audience. Correspondingly, these are the ones that have the highest potential to be harmed. Historically, learning best practices has occurred with, or at the expense of, women and birthing people.

Ever since birth moved out of the home and into the hospital at the turn of the century, providers have been attempting to replicate a normal physiological human process in one of the most extraordinarily nonphysiological manners. Many times, it works. Other times it doesn't work well. Sometimes it downright fails. Human labor is a process, though studied extensively, and has too many variables, too many predictors, too many moments of possible interjection to possibly know exactly how the process will unfold for any given individual at any given time. Human labor and birth remain the greatest unpredictable human function to this day.

Today, it would be unheard-of to see a birth occurring how it did even a few decades ago. However, from the 1950s, the upward trend of hospital births in favor of a more medicalized approach persisted alongside laws and regulations and obstructions making it difficult, and often illegal, to practice midwifery for the Black Southern traditional midwives, and difficult for other rural midwives to practice without having a formal education from a midwifery institution. By 1964 vital statistics records showed that of the 3,834,334 births that occurred in hospitals or institutions, 97.4 percent were delivered by physicians. The remaining 0.1 percent were delivered by midwives (CDC, *Vital Statistics of the United States*, 1970, vol. 1, Natality. 1975). Before midwifery was all but eradicated, the 1960s brought about some important groundwork as several midwives with higher educations were often trained OB nurses. These midwives established midwifery organizations and small cohort-type schools to help maintain the very small but steady growth of midwives.

It was in the 1970s at the resurgence of the so-called feminist movement where we noted a measurable shift in the location of birth and options for pregnancy and birth attendants. Women were being encouraged to embrace and normalize their form, function, and biology in ways that were previously unheard of. Autonomy of the

body was a right that was being demanded for its return. The outcomes of this movement poured over into a fight for reproductive rights and autonomy over when,
where, how, and with whom one chooses to labor and birth. Midwives were a perfect
fit into the feminist movement, as historically the embracement of labor and birth
as a normal human process were midwives' core tenets. Meanwhile, the South, still
reeling from the backlash of laws that restricted midwifery practice in conjunction
of a post–Jim Crow era, found that African American midwifery was pushed still
further underground and midwives continued to care for persons in their communities that were unable to receive care elsewhere. In some states such as Georgia,
Alabama, and Mississippi, midwifery was extinguished entirely. In the throes of the
American feminist movement of the 1970s is when midwifery decidedly and mea-
surably transitioned into what one might describe as nearly exclusively a white hip-
pie feminist movement. At this time, other types of midwives also continued to
persist. To make massive generalizations, they were Appalachian rural mountain
midwives, midwives that persevered in secluded religious sects throughout the
country, a very small number of hospital-based midwives, and the Black Belt Southern midwives, who straight through the late 1990s risked jail many times to provide
care to those who chose an out-of-hospital labor and birth with a midwife, while
their state laws decreed it to be illegal to practice midwifery. These exact same but
very separate veins of American midwifery continue in undercurrents to this day.

The respective growth of midwives along each type of midwifery continued at
their own pace, while some routes such as apprenticeship were stagnant, and others
such as traditional midwifery were nearly extinguished. Through the backdrop of
the feminist movement, throughout the intersections of the civil rights movement,
through social epidemics, through wars and presidents, through administrations,
through legislation, through health crises and even a couple pandemics, midwives
have maintained their presence in most places. By the 1980s midwives began to establish more politically influential organizations to more closely regulate the profession with minimum education requirements. Some of these organizations pushed
legislatively for the ability to prescribe medications and for independent practice.
By this time many paths of midwifery were nursing-based and had college and uni-
versity requirements for those not in an apprentice-learning model of midwifery. By
the 1980s and '90s, many of these organizations flourished alongside the growth of
hospital-based collaborative midwifery practices, as hospital-based midwives were
recognized and compensated as advanced-practice providers. Ultimately the primary driver for hospital-based births has always been the options for anesthesia for

pain control. Insurance reimbursements, the ability to find a provider, and ability to handle higher-risk labor and birth all ultimately pushed birth firmly into primarily hospital spaces. In 2020, 98.6 percent of births are planned hospital births. We also began to witness in 2020 our next shift.

Standing at the precipice of the COVID pandemic, birth visuals began populating the internet streets, providing views of labor and birth as something far different than it was even a generation ago. It is still a paradox. On one hand we see visuals of new parents, their faces behind masks, maybe in an operating room, and sometimes the fourth or fifth people to greet their newborn for the first time. Other visuals we have seen in the times of COVID have been an act of rebellion against the norm, exemplifying one's surefootedness in their decision to stay away from hospitals or to greet their babies in an out-of-hospital spaces. We are witness to birth being done in other ways, normalizing all the ways that we have been told labor and birth must be accomplished. Labor is something we do, not something that is done to us. Options are now seen as the standard. We are increasingly educated consumers. People want more, and people are demanding more. We have come a long way from when women were recovering from the grim picture that twilight birth brought.

Right now, the system of obstetrics is in one of those cycles or seasons of it not working as well as it could. One way we can tell when a system isn't working well is when we start to see disparities in outcomes for people who have babies. The thought is, since there aren't biological differences from one social political construct (race) to another, then there shouldn't be differences in birthing outcomes. Unfortunately, in the most recent tabulations (CDC, *Vital Statistics*) over the last decade, we find that Black women have an obstetric mortality rate that is on average three to four times the rates of non-Hispanic white women. Aside from this meaning that this obstetric system is not working as equitably as it could, this also leads to some questions that I think about often. Where in the stream of time did this system go wrong? When we find the place where there was a shift in how things started to have unfavorable outcomes, is there an opportunity for us to pause and redirect? I also wonder why some folks get so hell-bent on continuing to trek down a path that is no longer serving us in a mutually beneficial way? Lastly, and probably most importantly, can we trace it back to a time when birth was done differently, and somehow combine this intuitiveness with the sciences and strategies that we have improved over the last half century to create more favorable outcomes? The answer to that last question is, Yes, we can! This melding of intuitiveness with the sciences and strategies that we have improved over the last half century to create more favorable outcomes is called midwifery. No rational person would contest the fact that through obstetrics, we've learned some very important ways to make the birth experience safe and satisfactory, both by utilizing the sciences and resources when needed, and opting out of higher-risk strategies when we don't need it. We also have the benefit of having access to the most up-to-date information at any given time. This approach would translate into better outcomes, more favorable outcomes, more equitable outcomes for people who have babies.

I suggest that we take a closer look at the history of what has brought us to this place, one where birth has become a product of what someone else would like another person to physically accomplish. I also suggest we further examine the times when we started the conversation with the expectation that pregnancy, labor, and birth were normal processes that occasionally needed some medical intervention. Understanding some of the history of birth can sometimes change the trajectory of how we personally decide to navigate through pregnancy, how we labor, and how we birth. Each generation gets to decide. Each birth story, the future of birth history.

Dr. Stephanie Mitchell is a certified nurse midwife and author of The First-Time Parent's Childbirth Handbook: A Step-by-Step Guide for Building Your Birth Plan. *She developed the "Intermittent Auscultation Checklist," which helps labor and delivery providers of medical-industrial complexes identify candidates for low-intervention labor and birth. Dr. Mitchell is building Birth Sanctuary Gainesville, which will be the first freestanding birth center in the state of Alabama to serve the rural and surrounding communities. Connect with her on Instagram @Doctor_Midfwife.*

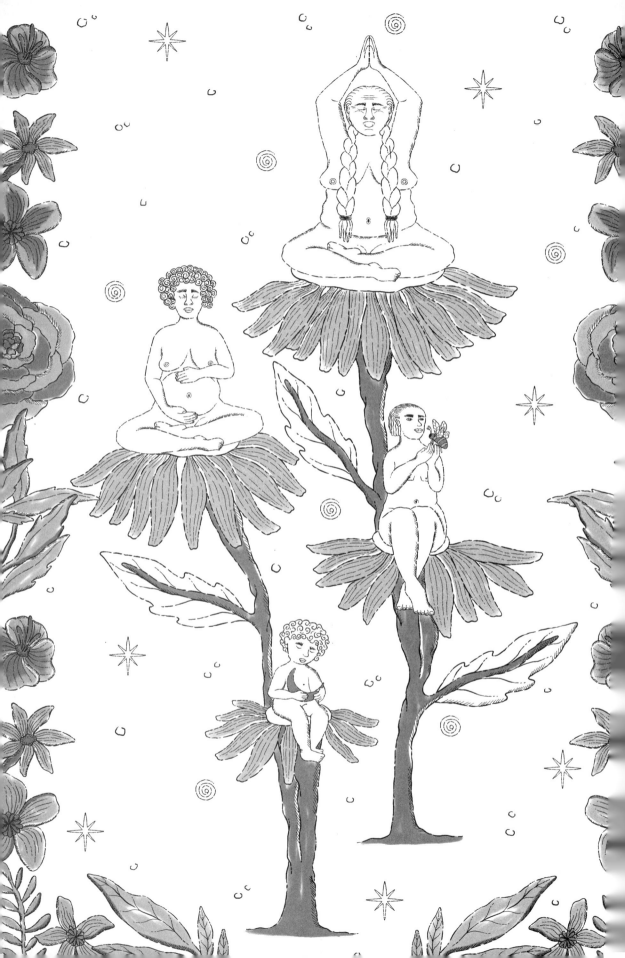

THE
EMBODIMENTS

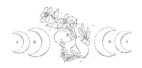

THE EMBODIMENTS

AN INTRODUCTION TO THE COURT CARDS

While it's probably possible to embody the energy of almost every card of the tarot, the Court Cards (traditionally named the Pages, Knights, Queens, and Kings) are the most accessible because they represent the energy of people, more so than a universal, disembodied archetypes like the Major Arcana represents.

I prefer the term *Embodiments*, because I try to be mindful to divest from hierarchies such as the royal court, but nonetheless in most decks these cards will be named that way: Page, Knight, Queen, King. For our purposes, another way to look at the energetic correlations of The Embodiments is infant, youth, parent, elder.

These cards can be read as an energy you're being called to step into. They can represent how someone else in your life is showing up for you, or because they are still complexly human, in some cases, they can indicate an energy of which to be wary.

The Pages are the youngest of the Embodiments, which give them a fresh and at times naïve energy. Their bright-eyed, awestruck nature hearkens to how we might feel about all the new sensations of pregnancy, and it also hearkens to the point of view our newborns will have of the world once they emerge and start discovering what it's like to be an earthling. The Pages are characterized as being inexperienced, but they make up for that in enthusiasm. I strongly believe in the necessity of our children bringing this energy to the world. We need imaginative thinkers who can see beyond what currently *is* and imagine what *could be*, becoming naïvely brave enough to make it happen. It doesn't hurt for us to inhabit this unjaded, fresh, imaginative energy of the Pages every now and then, too, so if a Page comes up in your spread, it might be a call to look at a situation with fresh eyes.

The Knights are the action-oriented "doers" of the Tarot, here to come in and check things off your to-do list. Their ambition pairs nicely with the Page's enthusiasm, so the two of them showing up in a reading and working together is a surefire way to see things through to completion. This is still a young and inexperienced energy, but similar to the Page, your outlook and approach have a lot to do with whether that's helpful or harmful. Naïveté is usually portrayed negatively, but considering how years of experience lead to apathy (how Kings can sometimes show up), experience isn't always necessarily a desirable attribute in pregnancy and birth either. The Knights help keep minds and opportunities open, bringing creative perspectives to problem-solving.

The Queens can represent maternal energy, but depending on the suit, that may or may not be expressed as nurturing. Queens are one of the two highest levels of achievement in each suit, which can give them a wise and experienced air. The Queens know what they're about and don't feel the need to please everyone. The Queens are crone-goals—whether they're able to offer the right amount of compassion without diminishing themselves or don't give a fuck about what people think about what they do or say. Queens are mature. They've lived through some shit. They don't engage in every drama that demands their attention. Their calm reserve doesn't come from not caring, it comes from having already lived through the vivacious ambition and enthusiasm of Pages and Knights and having already learned those lessons.

The Kings can represent paternal energy and can be benevolent, generous, and protective, or stingy, set in their ways, and cold. Kings are the other one of the two highest levels of achievement within the suit, which, when healthily expressed, can give them a stable, reassuring air. As pertains to pregnancy and birth, the energy that you might want to interrogate is when the Kings are showing up as controlling, punitive, dictatorial, dismissive, unemotional, and detached—these are all expressions of the Kings that frequently interfere with birthing folks' experiences during birth and postpartum (whether the King represents a family member, a care provider, or a partner).

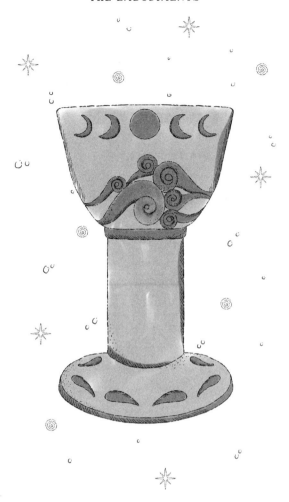

PAGE OF CUPS

The Page of Cups is bright-eyed and open to feeling new experiences without any guards up around their vulnerability. This can be interpreted as naïve, but when we're called into inhabiting this energy, in full recognition of the statistics, the possible hardships, the "what ifs," it's very brave. In a world that can feel like offense or defense are our only two options of being, softness, openness, and curiosity in the face of the unknown are revolutionary concepts.

What would the world, your pregnancy, your birth look like if you put on your "wonderment" goggles and let yourself be in awe of the sensations you're experiencing, both new and familiar? What would it look like to make your choices in pregnancy, birth, and postpartum from that place of curiosity instead of (perceived positive or negative) expectation?

OCEAN VISUALIZATION

If it feels safe and accessible to you, lie back, and imagine the sensation of floating in the ocean. Or better yet, if it's accessible to you, go float in a body of water! Let the water carry the weight of your belly for you; it'll feel glorious on your lower back. Yes, there are creatures inhabiting that ocean as well that, if your paths happen to intersect, could possibly do you harm. What now? You might sense that reality, get the heebie-jeebies, and flail about to find the quickest way out of the water, back to where your feet know stability and you can clearly see your surroundings. But if we're taking the medicine of the Page of Cups into account, particularly with birth in mind, we would stay and keep floating. We would surrender to the float with curiosity about what it feels like for our feet to be ungrounded, what it feels like to have a long, encompassing water hug. We would float with recognition that millions of people have floated in these exact waters, only to be embraced, held, and safe, coming out unharmed by any of the realities that inhabit the waters with us. See if you can access the childlike wonder that the Page of Cups shares with us as you rest and float. Treat each sensation as if it were the first time you ever felt it—maybe it actually is the first time you've felt the sensations you're feeling right now.

The freshness, wonder, and awe of this energy is one of the things we live for. And whether we acknowledge it or not, it's the sensation we're chasing when we decide to embark on the new experience of human making. Live into it with trust and faith.

ᖗ PAGE OF CUPS THEMES ᖘ
letting go, trusting, childlike curiosity, youth, fresh eyes

KNIGHT OF CUPS

No matter how far you are into your pregnancy or postpartum, this has been an emotional journey. And whether conscious, or unconscious, you've learned some ways to protect your vulnerabilities. That could manifest as choosing not to share your birth plan with certain people or being very discerning about who you'll allow into your space postpartum. This is ultimately a good thing. The cups are an emotional suit, and the Knight is action-oriented, here to protect those tender vulnerabilities, but it is capable of doing so with a loving, positive energy.

What's being called for in this card is to embody the lovable, positive energy of the Knight of Cups to firmly put up those protections (if you have not done so already) by way of making your boundaries and desires verbally clear. Doing so from a heart-centered place will be the best way to utilize this energy, so drop in and let your emotions lead this time. What you determine to be your boundaries around your pregnancy, birth, and postpartum don't need to be "logical" or approved by the overculture.

Inversely, if you have already set those boundaries and taken measures to protect your space and your emotional body during pregnancy and postpartum, then this card might be pointing out that you developed a hypervigilance when you initially set your boundaries. If this is the case, then this energy is letting you know it's safe to ease up a bit on your protective measures and open your heart up to a few select safe people who could potentially nourish you.

Be cautious not to let the energy of the Knight of Cups arise in an *I just want to get on to the next phase of this thing* kind of way. While this card is ambitious and therefore capable of enacting change and getting things done, it can also manifest as impatient and rob us of the sweet, more subtle experience of the Page. Pregnancy, birth, postpartum, and raising a human is not a series of checklists to get over with.

⊰ KNIGHT OF CUPS THEMES ⊱

energy, actionable steps, checking things off your to-do list, protecting yourself, ambition

QUEEN OF CUPS

You are being called to embody fluidity, both in your emotional body and your physical body. Rigid things are more likely to break. During pregnancy, the hormone relaxin will be softening the muscles in your round ligaments, loosening their grip on your pelvis in preparation to soften and be open.

During birth, softening your jaw and hands and surrendering to the intensity instead of fighting back will assist in opening your cervix, and in how you perceive the sensation of intensity. This card asks us to see what strength there is in softness and flow. You need only to go to a body of water or watch a thunderstorm to see the power inherent in flowing water. But if neither of those visuals are available to you, know that you literally are a walking (or sitting) body of water, and there is just as much power and strength within you as there is in the ocean.

The contractions of the uterus during labor are often described as "surges" or "waves," which is an accurate depiction. You see it coming in the distance; the undertow pulls at your legs, threatening to knock you over before the crest of the wave is even upon you. It might feel huge, too huge. Your eyes might widen at the enormity preparing to wash over you. You can flow or you can flail. You can surrender or you can fight. The Queen of Cups is a masterclass in choosing to *flow*.

⊰ QUEEN OF CUPS THEMES ⊱

a teacher for birth, flow, emotional intelligence, riding the wave, surrender, nurturance, softening

KING OF CUPS

The energy of the King of Cups is to either embody or call in the people with whom you feel like you can be your most open, authentic self. This energy makes a great addition to any birth team because they lead from a compassionate heart and clearly feel most at home in giving, which makes you feel comfortable receiving from them. You can easily find yourself crying in front of people who carry King of Cups energy because you know your full spectrum of emotions is in a safe, knowing place with someone who has this level of emotional intelligence. They aren't going to misplace it or pathologize it, just act as a steady container for it.

The King of Cups, when inhabited by a balanced, emotionally healthy person, makes everyone they encounter feel instantly safe without much effort on their part. The King of Cups, when inhabited by a person who is not appropriately introspective, who is only living from a place of their wounding, has the potential to be manipulative with their generosity and come off as very hot and cold.

You may be called to fulfill this role by reparenting yourself with compassion and unconditional love, all the acceptance and validation that you needed as a child. Or you may be called to lean on the people in your life who embody the positive attributes of this energy, knowing that you are safe and welcome to be embraced by them. It can also be a call to be cautious of the folks in your life who inhabit this energy only sporadically and on a good day, as this energy can be present in off-and-on, hot-and-cold partners of care providers.

⊰ KING OF CUPS THEMES ⊱

reparenting yourself, inner-child healing, emotional intelligence, introspection

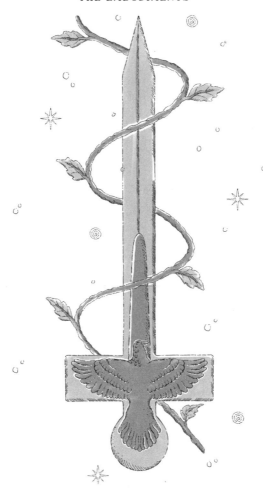

PAGE OF SWORDS

The Page of Swords energy is great for getting projects started, whether it's building your registry, planning a baby celebration, curating your nursery or baby space, or writing your birth plan.

Or maybe you inhabited this energy before you even conceived, reading all the books and preparing for pregnancy very proactively. The latter, while a beautiful and a noble endeavor, can be a sign that we are trying to prepare ourselves out of ever having to experience the hard lessons that are sure to come in pregnancy and birth. Prepared is good, but so prepared that you aren't still a humble student at the feet of this experience is a fast track to having a very humbling, knock-you-on-your-ass pregnancy, birth, or postpartum journey.

There's a lot of enthusiasm in this energy, but from a Page of Swords place, a quick way to suck the enthusiasm out of any project is to be too much of a perfectionist about it from the start. Recognize when you're just a beginner at something, and don't let perfectionism skew your perception of something that previously excited you.

Inversely, this energy can be a warning about being too pessimistic. When you're doing your research for making decisions around your birth location and birth plan, remember that you can find statistics and research to support anything. Beware of the pessimism or apathy that can come with the contradictory duality of information that's out there. The Page of Swords will want to get just the choices "right," in a cut-and-dry way, but pregnancy and birth is just not that simple. At some point, you're going to have to let your intuition have a say.

☽ PAGE OF SWORDS THEMES ☾

academic curiosity, research, becoming an expert in pregnancy and birth, prone to perfectionism, being proactive

KNIGHT OF SWORDS

The Knight of Swords has an innovative mind and all the confidence in the world to back that up. So much so that they can feel as if it isn't necessary for them to pause to reflect, second-guess themselves, or ask for a second opinion. In this way, the energy can easily show up imbalanced, so as helpful as this energy can be intellectually and for problem-solving, the Knight needs a more emotional counterpart to balance out their tendency to be cold, factual, or inhuman.

In pregnancy, this could show up as a partner, a helper, or even yourself, and the message is to bring in a more watery or grounded second opinion. The innovative potential of this card can break barriers and get you off the path of the status quo, or it can barrel you forward along the well-trodden path without ever even entertaining the notion that there are other options.

Consult someone with a perspective entirely different from your own, not necessarily because you need to change your mind about something, but because the Knight of Swords can be one-track-minded. This energy wants to barrel ahead without taking the time to ensure those checks and balances, but this intelligent, ambitious, get-it-done energy can be utilized in a helpful way only if you do the work to make decisions from a well-rounded place.

⸙ KNIGHT OF SWORDS THEMES ⸙

*making a plan, getting shit done, setting wheels in motion,
innovative thinking, problem-solving*

QUEEN OF SWORDS

Let me share with you a story about one of my favorite herbs, motherwort, to describe Queen of Swords energy: Motherwort has the energy of generosity, abundance, and nurturance. This is evidenced by her ease of propagating in less-than-ideal growing conditions and the medicinal benefits of working with motherwort for preparing for fertility, soothing anxiety, tending to the heart, lowering blood pressure, and treating postpartum mood disorders. It's the herb I reach for when I just want a hug from my mom. This is the herb I offer all postpartum people, whether it's the dried herb in sitz bath tea (see page 116) or tinctured to tend to the mood intensity of those early postpartum days (or trying toddler years).

At peak season, motherwort blooms little purple flowers, and the little spiky balls that grow up her stem are soft and welcoming to anything that chooses to land on her flowers and drink from her abundance. I would call this version of motherwort the pregnant version. Once motherwort goes to seed, however (postpartum motherwort), there is an entirely different vibe.

Once she dries, those spikes along her spine harden and they hurt if you touch 'em! Safe inside each little section there are four black seeds—her babies, what she'll leave behind.

The generous, welcoming Earth Mother energy is replaced by protectress, boundary queen, don't-fuck-with-me-or-my-babies energy in her postpartum season. Behind her painful boundary of spikes, her seed babies are safe from birds or anything else that would want to eat them. Eventually the seed babies will get shaken to the ground by wind and hopefully root into the ground on their own.

But interestingly, long after those spikes are empty of seed, motherwort stays hardened. The boundaries created during the postpartum season are often irrevocable.

Both seasons of motherwort are representative of the Queen of Swords archetype: nurturing and generous, overprotective and ruthless.

During pregnancy, the Queen of Swords is a beautiful energy to call upon when you need to advocate for yourself or call in your advocates to show up for you. You do not need to apologize for your decisions—your choices deserve to be honored and respected without explanation.

The Queen of Swords can give us intuitively clear-cut choices, which makes this a beautiful energy to call upon when writing your birth plan and when you are staking your boundaries and needs during your postpartum period.

Depending on your life circumstances and what experiences or traumas you're bringing to the table in pregnancy and birth, the Queen of Swords can also represent hypervigilant and fear-based choices (the hardened, spikey, overprotective "postpartum" version of motherwort).

These choices might seem practical or like "the only way" because fear and anxiety might be normalized experiences in your daily life. Do not judge yourself if you intuit that this is the way the Queen of Swords is showing up in you. There are hundreds of reasons in this lifetime and ancestrally that have injected fear and the assumption of incapability into the decision-making of pregnant people. To be influenced by that conditioning is entirely understandable and human. To be protective and spikey *is* valid and logical. Make room for softness amid the ruthlessness as well.

If this version of the Queen of Swords is what feels resonant, then honor this hypervigilant voice in your head and thank it for trying to protect you and your baby. This voice has done work to keep you safe at one point in your life. But that voice of hypervigilance and fear-based decision-making is never the most reasonable guide for the journey.

☽ QUEEN OF SWORDS THEMES ☾

protective, mama bear energy, acting from our wounding, impenetrable boundaries, hypervigilance, can sometimes be emotionally cold, can be too logical

KING OF SWORDS

When I think of the King of Swords, I think of a writer from whom I've learned so much, Kimberly Seals Allers.

In Dr. Stephanie Mitchell's chapter on the History of Birth in the US (page 125), you've seen the statistics that medical racism carried out by biased care providers is one of the largest contributing factors to the health disparities of Black birthing folks' experiences. Kimberly recognized this trend and created an app called Irth (*Birth without the B for Bias*) as a means for BIPOC to review their experiences at different hospitals and with different care providers. Kimberly went beyond recognizing that her community is not being served by the medical-industrial complex paradigm and created an entirely new structure of accountability. This kind of "building your own seat at the table" energy is what's possible in the King of Swords, and it does so in a tangible way that gets shit done and doesn't just dream about it.

Call upon this energy to figure out paperwork things like insurance. And if insurance doesn't cover the type of care you desire, the energy of this card doesn't take no for an answer and knows how to set up the crowdfunding campaign to fund it.

In a relationship, this can show up like every time you tell your partner about a pregnancy-related ailment you're experiencing, or emotion you're feeling, and they rush to "fix" it or see what they can do about it, instead of simply letting you express your feelings and difficulties. It's unlikely that they'll change that part of themselves at this point in the suit of swords, but take solace in knowing that trying to help in tangible (if sometimes cold) ways is how they show their love.

ᘓ KING OF SWORDS THEMES ᘔ

good at tasks that require mental capacity, filing paperwork, getting your affairs in order, practical solutions to problems, thinking bigger

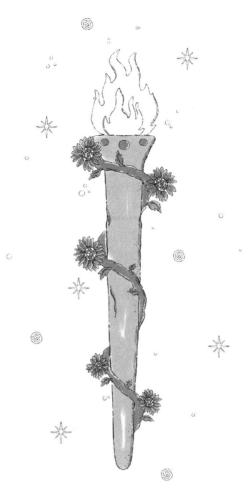

PAGE OF WANDS

I think of Page of Wands energy as the experience of doing a lot of research about pregnancy and birthing, being enthusiastic about what you've learned, and feeling resolute that the decisions you've made for your pregnancy and birth are deeply aligned.

Some people who perceive this energy in you will often want to remind you that you are new to this, that you aren't an expert, that Google doesn't make you a doctor. The truth or not of these kinds of responses is irrelevant, because the intention behind them isn't to help you as a birthing person but to disempower and diminish the bright-eyed and optimistic resolve of this Page. Luckily, when you're inhabiting the Page of Wands, naysayers tend to only add fuel to the fire, and the Page's truth just burns brighter, as if opposition is oxygen to their flame. And the truth is that you are the only person who has lived in your body your entire life, which makes you a valid, consultable expert on your own body and its care.

This is the type of person who often turns their pregnancy and birth experience into getting their doula certification, or eventually goes out for their midwifery education, or any other kind of professional modality around pregnancy and birth. The Page of Wands says, *Oh I'm not an expert? Watch me, bitch. I'll become one.*

ꙩ PAGE OF WANDS THEMES ꙩ
creativity, free spirit, having something to prove, believing in yourself

KNIGHT OF WANDS

The Knight of Wands takes the spark of fire and passion from the Page and puts it into motion with a Knight's actionable energy, which is helpful in achieving your goals.

Any inklings or callings that you might've heard as a whisper in the Page might be loud enough to act on now. If the path to or in parenthood has ignited a fire in you, fan it. If you're feeling called to a profession you previously didn't know existed but could see yourself contributing to now, start researching what kind of classes might be right for you to expand your interest into expertise.

There's a lot of potential when we're inhabiting this energy, and what's called for is to balance it out with honest vulnerability and focusing the flame. There are a lot of things to consider when you're pregnant and planning for birth. This energy is most helpful when you utilize it on one thing at a time, knowing that there is time for everything and that what's meant for you won't pass you by.

If you're working to make your pregnancy and birth aligned with the greater movement toward reproductive justice, then there are many avenues that you could go down because Black and Indigenous birth workers have been doing that work and building that legacy for centuries. Listen to and follow the lead of the voices who have been historically and currently most pushed to the margins by the white-supremacist patriarchy, as they aren't new to this.

No matter what level of knowledge you're starting with, there is a lot to learn, and this card is a reminder to focus your fire, especially if you are planning on directing that fire toward effecting change.

ꙩ KNIGHT OF WANDS THEMES ꙩ
ambitious, being fired up, intensity, being led by your passions, focus this energy, look to the elders for direction

QUEEN OF WANDS

This is one of my favorite energies to call upon during labor and birth. The Queen of Wands is at the pinnacle of a fiery, creative, sexual experience, and in birth, so are we. Our body's creative art project is ready to be shared, and it works in our favor to tap in both to inner fire and sensuality to birth them forth into the world.

The sensual nature of birth has been suppressed because of puritanical, patriarchal influence, and the Queen of Wands comes to remind us that you can be both parent and sexual being. This Queen is unapologetic about inhabiting both roles as a wholly nuanced human.

It comes very naturally to the Queen of Wands to lead by example and set the tone for the kind of care they expect in a birthing space, so this energy makes a great doula or birth support person. It is a great energy to call upon and embody during labor. Everyone in the room is there to serve and support *you* as the laboring person.

If it feels safe to you, ask for what you want/need without apology, set boundaries within your birth space, and take up the kind of space (physically and energetically) that you need. If you need to be sensual, be sensual. If you need to dance, dance. If you need to be alone, everyone has to go. If you need to roar, roar. If you need to sing, sing your baby earthside.

ᕁ QUEEN OF WANDS THEMES ᕤ
the pinnacle of creative potential, creative mastery, inhabiting sexuality,
sensual, unapologetic, self-assured

TAROT SPREAD FOR CALLING SENSUAL COMMAND INTO YOUR BIRTH SPACE

Find the Queen of Wands in your deck, and place it at the center of your spread. Then pull four cards for each of these questions:

What do I need to prepare in order to birth in total power?

What specific support do I need to call in?

What challenges or obstacles can I expect?

What message can bolster me in feeling confident about my birth?

KING OF WANDS

This energy is representative of someone who is powerfully influential. But influence, often combined with charisma, has the potential ability to also be manipulative, especially when this energy is inhabiting an unhealthy expression, or when someone with this energy is not vigilantly seeking accountability.

I think of this energy as being signified by some of the educators and care providers in birth, spirituality, and even social justice movements. Sometimes the people who hold the most influence or have the biggest platform to be heard are out of touch with the needs of everyday people. In tarot language, sometimes once we've reached the King of Wands, we forget the little spark that lit the Ace of Wands.

If this card is showing up as another person in your spread, it's time to dig in and find the underrepresented story or stories that might be opposing or overshadowed by the King of Wands' ray of influence.

If this card is showing up as representative of you or an energy you need to embody, then it is pointing to the immense creative life force you have available within you. This is a powerful, helpful energy particularly at the height of birth's intensity. Stepping into this energy for ourselves particularly in the creative act of birth is when we get to meet the enormity of our magical potential face-to-face. This is such a potent energy that harnessing it requires a very careful balance.

A birthing person who is embodying the King of Wands is going to need a very respectful, quiet birth team that knows what to do without asking, a birth team that tends to all the senses (therapeutic sounds, smells, physical touch, soft lighting). As a birthing person, the King of Wands needs birth to be a ritual. So, the team needs to know how to make the ideal space for the birthing person to "go there," to tap into that transcendent, almost otherworldly power to bring their creative life force into the world.

KING OF WANDS THEMES

remember why you started, stay grounded, being in command, ultimate creative potential

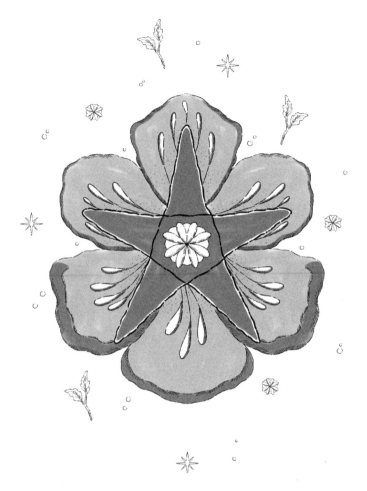

PAGE OF PENTACLES

The Page of Pentacles is like the energy of a person who goes into pregnancy trying to be a "good pregnant person" and gets everything right. This energy might even have a little bit of a complex where they put their care provider on a pedestal or have "white coat syndrome"* around their OB.

This is the kind of energy where one routinely gives their power away by structuring their lifestyle and decision-making around what their doctor will or won't "allow" during pregnancy and birth. While I'm sure plenty of people have satisfactory birth experiences from this conventional, status-quo-upholding place,

....

* White coat syndrome is when your blood pressure reads higher at the doctor's office than when you are at home or in an otherwise relaxed space. "White coat" refers to the color of clothing most doctors wear, but it generally means being put on edge by someone you've deemed as a medical authority figure.

ultimately those paradigms are rooted in a white-supremacist patriarchy. This type of energy assumes that what the patriarchal medical-industrial complex has decided as "safest and best" is the only way of birthing a baby, which erases midwifery knowledge because that wisdom is held matriarchically by Black and Indigenous birth workers.

I would challenge anyone who sees this energy in themselves to dig deeper than conventional wisdom—because you have to dig only about a hundred years to find that there's nothing normal about what we consider "normal" in birth these days. Why do things by the book when the proverbial "book" was not written with BIPOC or even the best interests of all people with uteruses in mind?

Ultimately, this card is a warning to not idolize any perceived authority figure above yourself. Not because you know everything and can't trust your team, but because there's no way out of building a relationship with and listening to your intuition. Your care providers are still potentially fallible humans. The people who did the scientific studies are still fallible humans. We've been getting birth wrong for decades, in some cases centuries, and despite new evidence, some birth care providers still practice non-evidence-based birth practices. The pedestal on which we put the medical-industrial complex is an unearned seat.

◁ PAGE OF PENTACLES THEMES ▷

trying to do everything "right," giving away your personal power to someone else,
discounting the value of your intuition, a call to empower yourself with
your own research and tapping into intuition

KNIGHT OF PENTACLES

In preparing for birth, the Knight of Pentacles comes in to remind us how to root down into the earth, remembering how one we are with the elements. Nearing the end of your pregnancy, leading up to birth, it's okay to be almost stubbornly grounded. As obligated as you may feel, now is not the time to be in your head, taking in new information, making new plans, or watching the news.

This energy makes an amazing meditation teacher, but if it's showing up as an energy for you to embody yourself, then you might need to be your own gentle guide.

Whenever you feel your mind wandering off, your ego creating stories, your brain wondering about the future (in either joy or anxiety) or anything else that gets you out of your body, take your physical body outside. If it's possible for the weather you have, or the area that you live in, remove your shoes and get your feet in contact with the earth. Ground yourself here for as long as you need to, slowly and methodically, feeling your roots reaching through your feet and deep into the earth. If eventually you get fidgety, place your hands on your hips and do some figure-eights. Try to stay in your body in this moment.

◁ KNIGHT OF PENTACLES THEMES ▷

staying rooted, moving your body, not allowing the thinking brain to
run rampant, grounding into your body

QUEEN OF PENTACLES

For some of us pregnant folks (not all, but some), this will be our quintessential idea of what parenthood is, because this is the "earth goddess" archetype. But whether that imagery aligns with our identity or not, the medicine of this card is a nourishing one.

If you are called to embody this energy yourself and don't know where to start, go outside into nature. You don't need an agenda for what to do while you're out there, but this energy is naturally inclined toward foraging plant medicine (ethically and safely), so if you know how to identify plants (if you don't, there are free apps for this), now is a good time to respectfully forage plant medicine like motherwort to support your mood postpartum or plantain leaf to dry for a postpartum sitz bath (see page 116).

If you're not feeling called to embody this energy yourself, or not right now, you can also call upon it during pregnancy and birth if you feel lost or scared or when doing inner-child work. The Queen of Pentacles is a loving parent energy, so it's especially useful to access if that's not something we had when we were children ourselves and we just want to be held. In fact, I'll go ahead and say for everyone for whom this card comes up—you are held right now, even if you're not feeling it in the ways you are used to perceiving things. (See Eight of Pentacles, page 94, for a guided visualization to facilitate this sensation of being held.)

Through this card, you could be called to reach out to a person in your life who has this kind of nurturing energy. Know that people who embody this energy are authentically generous and enjoy abundance themselves, so giving freely comes naturally to them. This means you don't have to feel guilty for taking up their time, crying on their shoulder, or letting yourself be held by this person. In fact, people with Queen of Pentacles energy live for being there in that nourishing, nurturing, unconditional kind of way. This is the friend or family member you want to invite to stick around with you in your immediate days and weeks postpartum.

◁ QUEEN OF PENTACLES THEMES ▷

ultimate nurturer, caretaker, who you're becoming but also who you need to be surrounded by, nourish and be nourished

ʙONE BROTH

Bone broth is one of the most nutritional foods for postpartum healing. It brings the warmth the body needs to restore after birth, as well as vitamins and minerals, protein, and collagen for replenishing the blood and repairing tissues. Even in a straightforward vaginal birth, it is still common to lose up to 500 ccs of blood. On top of that, your baby just subsisted on and took up the nutrients in your body for nine months, and if you are feeding your baby from your body, then that nutrient supply continues to be drained. Replenishing vitamins and minerals is essential postpartum, as is keeping your protein intake up just as you did in pregnancy.

I suggest making this ahead of time and then keeping it in your freezer to thaw whenever you're ready for it.

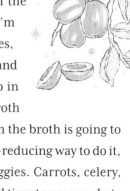

Truthfully, you can make bone broth from just bones and water; everything else is to either add more nutrients or more flavor. Whenever I'm lucky enough to have bones, my partner already knows to make space in the freezer because I'll be making broth! Every time I'm prepping veggies, I toss all the scraps—the pepper cores, carrot tops, potato peels, artichoke leaves, onion tops and skins, cilantro stems—in a resealable bag that I keep in the freezer at all times. This is what I use to flavor broth whenever I'm ready to make it. Everything brewing in the broth is going to get strained out anyway. That's the economical, waste-reducing way to do it, but you can also use whole cleaned and chopped veggies. Carrots, celery, and onions are common soup flavors, but now is a good time to use up whatever veggies you have in the refrigerator.

This recipe is highly customizable and ancestral. Don't get caught up on the measurements or worrying over not having certain ingredients. Work with what you have; it will be enough. And a whole lineage of grandmothers will be smiling upon you through the veil for your efforts.

INGREDIENTS

Bones (such as chicken, beef, oxtail, turkey—whatever you have on hand)

Vegetables or vegetable scraps (such as carrots, celery, onions, winter squashes, dried mushrooms—whatever you have on hand; optional)

Red dates (optional)

Fresh herbs (such as thyme, rosemary, lemongrass, sage; optional)

Dried nutritional herbs (such as nettles, oat straw, alfalfa, red raspberry leaf; optional)

Sea salt

EQUIPMENT

Large stockpot

Fine-mesh strainer

INSTRUCTIONS

You can roast your bones in the oven first for richer flavor, if you'd like. Just coat them in olive oil, put on a baking sheet, and roast at 400°F for 30 minutes or until they brown.

Transfer the bones to a large stock pot, cover with water completely, add your veggies, dates, and herbs, if desired, and bring it to a boil. Once boiling, immediately turn the heat down to a low simmer. Allow the broth to simmer on low, uncovered, for 8 to 12 hours.

Strain out the bones, veggies, and herbs with a cheesecloth or fine-mesh strainer. Add sea salt to taste.

The broth can be drunk immediately or stored in glass jars in the refrigerator or freezer (allow glass jars to cool completely before freezing).

KING OF PENTACLES

If you pulled the King of Pentacles as representative of yourself, then you are likely going to feel most at ease during pregnancy, birth, and postpartum by being resourceful enough to meet your own needs. This energy is used to having enough, needs to know there will be enough, and is very thrown off by the possibility of there not being enough. This could be the idea of not enough financial resources, not enough community connections, not enough support for postpartum, and so on. But getting those ducks in a row is going to be what makes the King of Pentacles feel assured.

It's not uncommon for this energy to show up in whoever is the partner to the pregnant person (if there is one). Dealing in the material preparations for birth and postpartum is the most readily available way for a partner to feel ready and prepared, since it's not their own body doing the physical preparations. Instead, they tend to deal with more of the material preparations, offering them one way they can feel useful.

I caution you against "doing too much." Do the things on your checklist to prepare but let that be enough. Creating more things to put on the checklist can be a never-ending method of taking ourselves out of the experience of pregnancy (whether you're the pregnant one or not), which is a way that our brains avoid letting the enormity of what's to come sink in. So, get done what you need to get done, yes, but then call upon this energy to root you back down into the body, into the earth, and be present with your current stage of pregnancy or postpartum.

ᚷ KING OF PENTACLES THEMES ᚱ

do less, busy hands are not always best, be in the moment, a calm reassuring presence, that person in your life who is your "rock"

ᴱEXERCISE

FOR PARTNERS
AT ANY PHASE OF PREGNANCY,
POSTPARTUM, OR PARENTING

I know that when your partner is the one doing all the human-growing, it can feel like the only way for you to contribute is with your hands—doing the tasks they don't have the energy for right now, maybe spearheading meal making and planning or attending to the practical, everyday tasks of preparing to be a parent or being a parent. As helpful and necessary as all those tasks are, it's an easy way for life to feel methodical and mundane. It's easy to lose ourselves when we inhabit this space too long.

Take a moment to ground yourself, wherever you are right now. Close your eyes. Nourish your body with three deep oxygenating belly breaths.

Now try to inhabit the brain of your twelve-year-old self (or whatever age comes to mind when you picture yourself as a kid). Now, when you open your eyes, pretend it's twelve-year-old you looking around.

What do they notice? What do they think about your partner? What do they think about you being a parent now? Look around your space. How does twelve-year-old you feel about where you live, the things that fill up your space, or pets you have?

Without judgment, take a moment to write down what words came to mind when you were looking at your life from your child-self's eyes: *gratitude, awe, disappointment, fear, pride, joy, neutrality—all feelings are welcome.**

---

* Shout out to my partner, Alex, for suggesting this practice that helps him stay grounded in the moment and feel gratitude for his life.

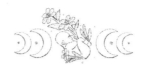

RESOURCES FOR FURTHER EXPANSION

These kinds of lists to expand upon your learning usually show up at the end of books, but I wanted to highlight these folks and any resources they may offer here, right before you dive into the Major Arcana. When you're preparing for pregnancy and parenthood, this book is one way to look at your experience but certainly does not stand alone. Understanding your birth and pregnancy journey requires additional, self-empowered research and actionable work to ensure you're showing up as the kind of parent you want to be on your path to and in parenthood.

Here is a list of books, people to learn from, podcasts, and other resources that enriched and improved my experiences in pregnancy and parenthood, and the world into which I'm choosing to bring another human.

- *Awakening Fertility* by Heng Ou is a great place to root your prepregnancy journey in nutrition and ancestral wisdom.
- *Real Food for Pregnancy* by Lily Nichols gives an updated look at nutritional guidelines for a whole foods–supported pregnancy.
- *Nurture* by Erica Chidi Cohen is an all-encompassing pregnancy guide from preconception to postpartum, detailing all the scientific and medical jargon that may or may not apply to your pregnancy.
- *The First-Time Parent's Childbirth Handbook* by Dr. Stephanie Mitchell, CNM, CPM, is a compact, inclusive guide to learning your options and crafting your birth plan from an informed place.
- *Me and White Supremacy* by Layla F. Saad is the challenge I accepted in 2018 when I decided to stop exceptionalizing myself as "one of the good

ones" and investigate the ways in which I am complicit in white supremacy. My son was a newborn at the time, and the realization that I was signing up to continue my family legacy was really beginning to sink in. I knew as a white person who would be raising a white-passing child that I was going to be ill-equipped on my own to speak to him on the topic of race and how white supremacy is woven into the fabric of our daily lives, and even more ill-equipped on what to do about it. It was and still is imperative to me that I did not prioritize my comfort or my own child's "innocence" at the expense of the comfort, innocence, and lives of Black folks, Indigenous folks, and every other person of color. If you're familiar at all with antiracism work, then you've probably heard that this work is lifelong, which is true. But for anyone who holds white privilege, Layla's book is an excellent place to start that work, recognizing that the work begins with us first.

- Leesa Renée Hall helps highly sensitive folks explore their implicit biases through her emergent "Inner Field Trip" work on Patreon. I have found her work to be integral to the "lifelong" aspect of continually noticing and rooting out biases, and Leesa achieves that through expressive writing prompts. Her work can be accessed on Patreon and www .leesareneehall.com.

- *The Altar Within* by Juliet Diaz is a magical book to reconnect you with your divine self and forge a more intimate connection with Spirit and your ancestors through self-worship.

- *Birthful*, a podcast by Adriana Lozada, is the most comprehensive pregnancy, birth, and postpartum resource I've come across. In this podcast you'll find evidence-based birth information, pregnancy nutrition information, newborn sleep information, explorations on the medical choices you'll make on behalf of your child, birth stories from real people, and so much more. If you have a partner, I recommend listening in the car on long drives so that you're learning together.

- *The First Forty Days* by Heng Ou is a beautiful guide to planning for a healing and protected postpartum period.

- *The Big Letdown* by Kimberly Seals Allers was an integral part of fully forming my education on breast/chestfeeding. While books like *Nurture* by Erica Chidi Cohen will cover the actual mechanics and science of feeding your baby, *The Big Letdown* will provide you with the necessary knowledge of the social mechanics and systemic barriers that will impact your breast/chestfeeding journey and inform your self-advocacy if you meet obstacles. At the time of my writing this book, Kimberly Seals Allers also has a prototype for an app called Irth (*Birth* without the *B* for *Bias*) to act as a database of hospital and care provider reviews to help empower pregnant folks' choice in care provider, inform them on their history, and start holding care providers accountable.

- *Tarot for the Wild Soul* is a podcast created by Lindsay Mack that will help expand upon and evolve your understanding of the tarot from a soul-led place. Lindsay also offers courses as well, for soul-centered tarot learning. Lindsay Mack's work can be found on www.lindsaymack.com.

- The Conscious Kid is an organization teaching and providing resources for parenting and education through a critical race lens. Their work can be accessed on Patreon and Instagram @theconsciouskid.

- To find a Black midwife, doula, lactation consultant, or wellness practitioner in your area, visit www.sistamidwife.com for a directory.

Throughout reading this book, you will see quotations highlighted (that were used with consent, reciprocity, and gratitude) from a trusted set of birthworkers, mystics, traditional practitioners, etc. I hope you'll explore the folks on the above list, and the folks who are sporadically quoted in this book, to find the voices that resonate with you to start building and rounding out a spirit team whose voices and wisdom will accompany you in this important journey of raising the next generation.

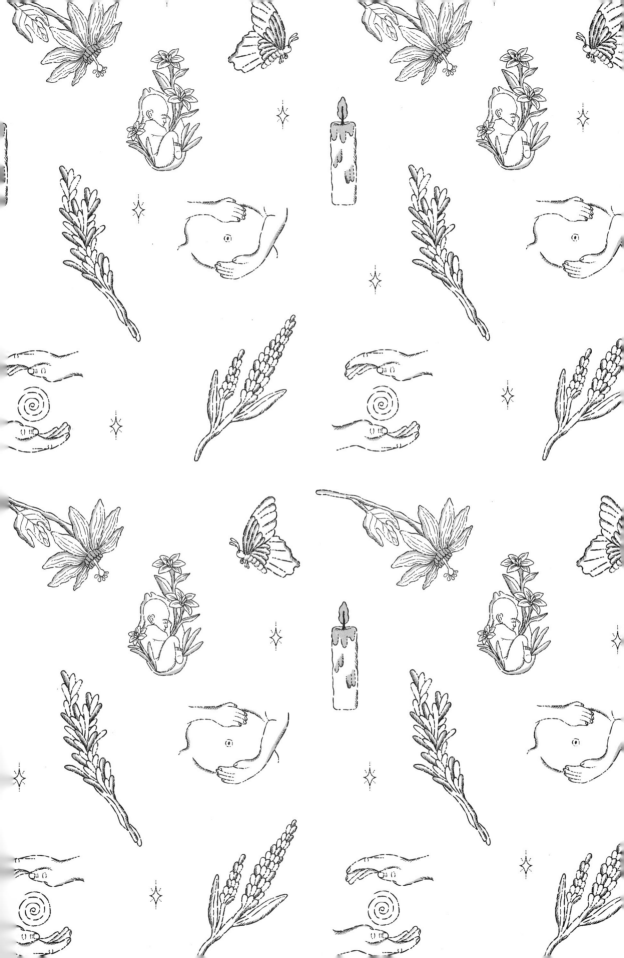

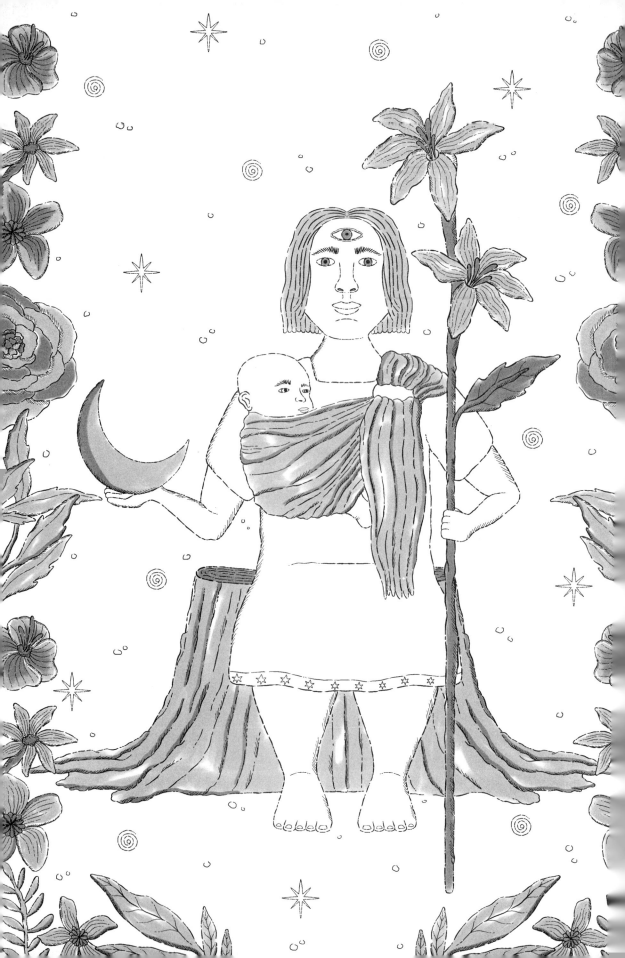

THE SOUL ARCHETYPES

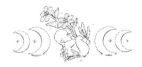

THE SOUL ARCHETYPES

In what's referred to as the Major Arcana, we find the big milestones everyone goes through in life, often more than once. Some of these are represented in typical tarot imagery by embodied archetypes (*embodied* meaning imagery centered on humans), but these are more realistically seen as energies that pass through us from time to time—not necessarily something that we are perpetually.

Sometimes these energies force themselves into our lives unwanted for the sake of our ascension, and sometimes they are energies we actively call in or happily welcome, also for the sake of our ascension. Unlike the daily, nitty-gritty, minutiae energy of the Minor Arcana, these energies are harder to ignore, because they're *big*, representing seasons and eras of our whole lives, not just what's going on that week or month. Because of that, it's not unusual to have whole spreads with no Major Arcana cards, indicating that what you're dealing in is a problem of the current moment but not necessarily a big life lesson.

This is also why whenever you are in an era where you're integrating the lessons of a specific soul archetype, you might find those Major Arcana cards repeating themselves in your spreads (see "A Note on Repeating Cards," page 21).

I'll also say that when Major Arcana cards show up in a spread, they are often an opportunity, something you can decide whether you want to reach for. As with all relationships, your consent also applies when it comes to your relationship with the divine and your ancestors, and they might be suggesting an opportunity for healing that you don't want to take them up on yet. These energies are *big*, and if you pass on their lessons at this time, they will surely make themselves available again when you might be more ready to receive their medicine, or when life events force you to learn their lessons.

You'll find there is a good amount of variation in chapter length in these coming chapters, and that's not me playing favorites with the cards, but simply because some cards hold more relevance to the parenthood path than others.

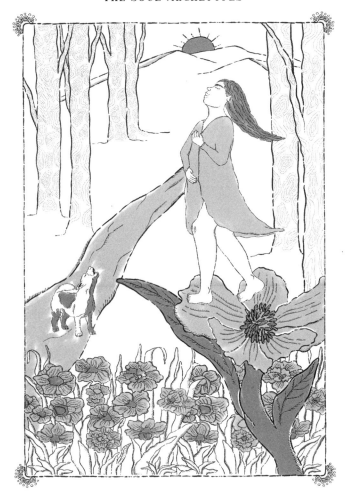

0—THE FOOL

In the Fool, we are diving into something headfirst, despite any warnings we've received, be they wise or misguided. We are moving ahead on the cusp of our journey, hopefully because something within tells us that the universe has a built-in safety net for us.

The Fool, much like attempting to create a new human, is one big leap of faith, putting our hearts and our dreams on the line, knowing that we have the possibility of being let down, knowing that we're making our hearts potentially vulnerable for the breaking.

Traditionally, in the Smith-Rider-Waite Tarot, artist Pamela Colman Smith depicts the Fool as a person taking unexamined steps forward, seemingly about to walk right off a cliff, with their dog at their feet barking, offering a warning about the imminent precipice in front of them that the fool is naïvely ignoring.

What that dog is barking at us will be different for each person who thinks they want to embark on the parenthood journey. For some of us experiencing life at different intersections of oppression, your metaphorical dog might be barking, *But the Amazon is on fire! CO_2 emissions are still on the rise with no game plan! How can you bring another carbon-footprint-having garbage maker into existence!?* For some of us experiencing life as a marginalized human, our dog might be barking, *This world won't be safe for your Black child! What about when they are no longer a cute baby but a young preteen who the world, with all its unchecked biases, sees as a threat? How could you bring another human into the world to experience the pain of racism, sexism, classism, homophobia, transphobia, or ableism?* For some of us, our dog might simply be barking, *But you don't have enough worldly resources to afford to care for yourself, let alone another human!*

This dog represents society and our cautious thinking brain, not the needs and desires of our soul's journey, nor the needs and desires of the soul that's trying to come back to Earth through you, arriving here to do what they were meant to do. This dog seeks to keep us safe but small. We can thank the dog (or our brain) for its trepidation, thank it for helping us survive this far, but ultimately, we should be giving more credence and authority to our intuitive desires and not our limiting fears.

The stubbornly persistent existence of white supremacy as the standard does not get to determine who gets a chance to experience parenthood. The inhumane, unrealistic, and ableist demands of capitalism should not get to gate-keep health, survival, or happiness like it currently does. The colonial and white-supremacist standard of what qualifies for a "civilized" life that has taxed our Mother Earth's well-being so detrimentally for the past few centuries should not get to dictate whether we choose to experience the parenthood journey (it is my personal belief that to do so is to already admit defeat in regard to the climate and the health of our Mother). We aren't continuing to have babies in spite of apocalyptic world circumstances, but precisely *because* of that. The world needs the fresh eyes, the emergent thinkers, the healing souls that are asking to come through right now.

So, what then? Do we just barrel ahead with our parenthood plans, pretending that those realities are not playing a real and valid role in our decision-making around whether to procreate? I sure hope not. Taking a look at the state of the world, and deciding that you want to create another human to exist in that world—not with the wool over your eyes about the reality of the climate (literal, political, and cultural) you'll be introducing them to—but stepping into the parenthood journey with bold, utter clarity and the knowledge that the humans you create and/or raise, how you choose to bring them into the world, and how you choose to raise them up, has the potential to shift culture, shift paradigms, shift narratives, and spark change.

In this way, we are stepping into this role of parent not in denial of reality, but in spite of and *because of* that reality with *intention and action* to create the changes we want to see in the cultural narrative. If you are someone who does want to be a parent, parenthood has the potential to be an enormous act of activism and hope.

⤜ THE FOOL THEMES ⤛

start of a journey, newborn, fresh eyes, bold naïveté, acting upon our decision, fertility, conception, refers to the Aces

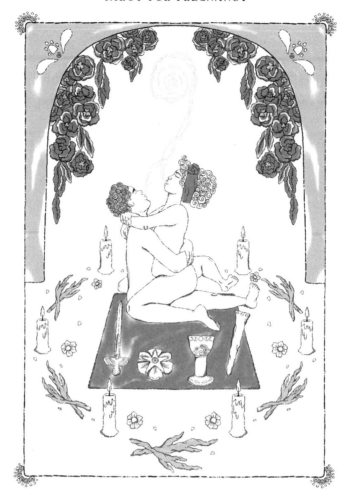

1–THE MAGICIAN

We all have the ability to tap into our inner Magician archetype, and the act of conception, pregnancy, and birth is just one very tangible expression of that. Within us, we have all that is needed for the building blocks of life. With the right ingredients, we can begin the alchemy of cell division that will eventually become the baby you birth. It's magic in one of its truest forms.

You can call upon Magician energy when you are trying to conceive, and once pregnant, you can call upon Magician energy to manifest the kind of birth experience you want. And I mean manifest in the way of recognizing your own power and taking up your own tools, not manifest in the traditional sense of controlling a certain favorable outcome.

The leap of faith into conception that the Fool took is picked up by the Magician who is now acting as a conduit for that creative energy. Because of this, traditionally the Magician can be an active "hit the ground running" energy after the Fool's leap into a new beginning; the Magician is where we actually start.

In pregnancy, especially right after conception, the task at hand is not necessarily to "do" much, at least not anything that looks like outward action. At this point, it's time to recognize and internalize that this power, this magic, this creative energy is in you, happening whether you notice it or not—but I truly hope you pause to start noticing it.

So, start getting comfortable with the idea that you have that power (Hint: You always have) and sensitize yourself to accepting just how fucking magical and powerful you are. This mindset will serve you throughout your pregnancy, into birth, and it will empower you in your parenting experiences too.

◁ THE MAGICIAN THEMES ▷

alchemy, tools at your disposal, the elements, having all the tools already in you,
making something out of nothing, practicing witchcraft,
mastery over your magic, creation

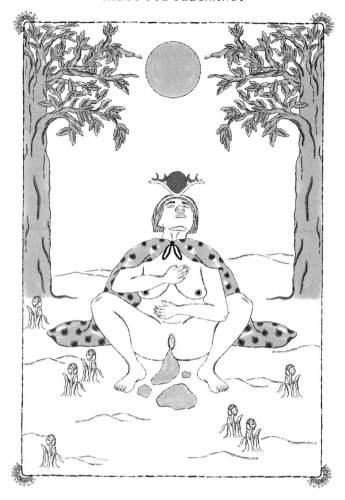

2–THE HIGH PRIESTESS

The High Priestess is the energy I prefer to invoke when I am not pregnant and trying to connect to my menstrual cycle. Ideally, this is the kind of connection you would make and relationship you would build with your cycle before you even try to become pregnant, so if you pull this card and you are not yet pregnant, then this is what's being asked of you: learn body literacy* in regard to your menstrual cycle and develop a spiritual connection to that cycle, however that looks for you.

The High Priestess has a strong connection with the moon (which is why it's common for imagery of the High Priestess in the tarot to include a moon), as does

---

* Body literacy is the practice of observing, learning, and understanding the distinctive processes of your body, particularly used in knowing the four phases of the menstrual cycle. Erica Chidi Cohen is an author and advocate I've learned from about the topic of body literacy.

menstruation: When you bleed corresponds with the new moon, the follicular phase (leading up to ovulation) corresponds with the waxing moon, ovulation (the release of an egg and the lining of the uterus to prepare for a potential wombmate) corresponds to the full moon, and then the luteal phase (preparing to nourish a fertilized egg, if there is one) corresponds with the waning moon. This is why it's common for a menstrual cycle to last twenty-eight days, the same length of the cycle of the moon.

I'm assuming that if you're reading this book, you or someone you love has a uterus and you or they are intending to try to grow a baby in said uterus. In which case, menstruation is highly applicable to pregnancy, both for the obvious physical reasons but also for noticing and connecting to the subtle ebbs and flows of one's monthly cycle.

There is a myriad of reasons why we shy away from body literacy or don't feel intimately involved with our menstrual cycle. Sometimes it's because we just don't even think to connect with it, maybe we think it's an annoying, unwelcome aspect of our bodies, or maybe we hold the false idea that to be connected with and knowledgeable about menstruation is a strictly feminine concept or female responsibility (it's not). I firmly believe in being knowledgeable about and loving toward our bodies (whether that's the body we were born with, or the body we choose to affirm what we know internally to be true). One of the lessons of the High Priestess is to build a relationship of respect and understanding with menstruation, if it's a physiological function that happens for you.

As a person who bleeds, one of the ways I honor my body's cycles is by tracking and knowing where I am in my cycle, so I can play into the corresponding moon-phase energies of that stage in the cycle (whether that be the rest and restore of a new moon, or the outward, sexual, creative expression of the full moon).

When I learned that menstrual blood has stem cells in it, it suddenly made sense to me why the patriarchy demonized menstruation and painted it to be a dirty waste product to be hidden away and never mentioned. The presence of stem cells in menstrual blood means there's big power in there, power that the patriarchy would not like us to know we wield. All blood is powerful, that's why blood is one of the most potent ingredients in magical workings, but menstrual blood is unique in that it requires no violent sacrifice to obtain.

For that reason, once I learned that, it's now part of my menstrual practice to try and not waste that potent tool for magic. I collect it, water it down, and use it to nourish the plants that grow around my home, speaking intention along with it, usually offering it back to the earth as an expression of gratitude and sacrifice (though it's more just a sacrifice of my time and convenience because, like I said, it doesn't require violence). It can also be used for protection magic or for a fertility ritual as a part of your conscious conception.

⇥ HIGH PRIESTESS THEMES ⇤

trusting yourself, inward reflection, unbothered, menstrual cycle, receptivity but with strong boundaries, divinity, recognizing divinity within yourself

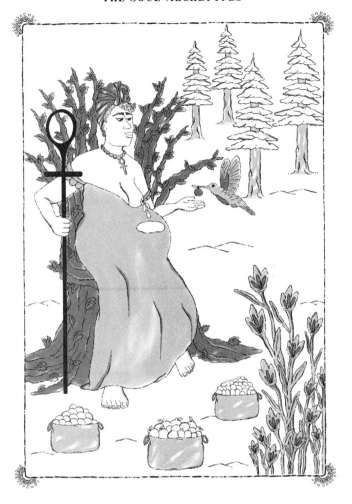

3—THE EMPRESS

"To be sensual, I think, is to respect and rejoice in the force
of life, of life itself, and to be present in all that one does,
from the effort of loving to the breaking of bread."
—James Baldwin, Black queer writer and activist

Societally induced shame around our bodies is one thing that can frame a feeling of
shame around our sexuality (which we will explore more once we reach the Devil
archetype, page 211). But there are also the traumas of past experiences that can and
will try to rise and have their say when you're needing to tap into a more primal
brainwave during pregnancy and birth.

I believe the matriarch of the tarot, the Empress, holds some comfort and wisdom in working through some of that trauma, enough to reclaim divine sensuality

for ourselves, not for anyone else. I think if we are attempting conception from this magical state of mind, we are setting ourselves up for a deeply meaningful and healing pregnancy experience.

The Empress is passion embodied, and they're unapologetic about their sexuality, too, which makes this an effective energy to call upon if you'll be increasing your chances of conception using sex magic. To be honest, I think all sex is magic (not always in a pretty way), which is how unplanned pregnancies can happen when portals are unknowingly opened through the act of intercourse.

But you can do more than that, especially if you're wanting to affect a certain outcome when it comes to the trajectory of your pregnancy and birth. Intentional, consensual sex magic is simply one way of raising the energy available to you at any given moment in order to add that energy toward manifesting a certain aligned outcome.

This can be solo, but if you do have a partner, make sure you communicate and obtain consent from them to utilize your sexual activity for magical purposes. You always need to obtain consent, not only for the obvious reasons when you're practicing magic on or with another person other than yourself, but also so you can have their intent too. Because sex magic is simply a way to raise energy to increase the chances of getting what you want (which in this case is to get pregnant or support a healthful vital pregnancy). It is still possible (and maybe even more useful) to consider utilizing the energy of sex magic even if you intend to become pregnant via IVF (as long as your doctor says that sexual activity is safe during treatments and fertilization).

The passion, sensuality, and unashamed irreverence of the Empress also makes this a beautiful nourishing energy to call upon to come home to your body and reclaim what your sexual expression uniquely means for you, whether you're trying to conceive or not or when you're already pregnant. This is going to look different for everyone, but ways to invite this energy in through lushness (plants, flowers), opulence (abundance of beautiful things, soft textiles), and prioritizing the earthly pleasures of your body (orgasms, fruit, chocolate, warm sun on your skin, plenty of sleep).

The environmental conditions of the Empress also happen to be the environmental conditions that promote birth, so this is a lovely energy to invoke during labor and birth. If you can't surround yourself with those things, then the Empress shows us how to see the beauty and abundance in places we wouldn't expect. The Empress teaches us how to receive and ask for help even if a previous version of ourselves wouldn't have been comfortable. The Empress doesn't need affirmation cards to know they are worthy and deserving of love, goodness, and abundance, they already naturally radiate that certainty.

The Empress is gentle and forgiving with the parts of you that are human and fallible, so we can learn from the Empress in this way and treat ourselves with that same grace as we learn to receive as much as we give.

◁ THE EMPRESS THEMES ▷

nourishment, the earth, parenthood, sensuality, full embodied sexuality, unapologetic indulgence, opulent abundance, the art of receiving

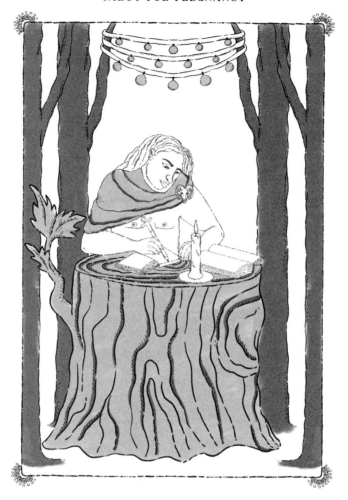

4-THE EMPEROR

"The power of a birth plan isn't the actual plan. It's the
process of becoming educated about all your options."

—unknown

When I think of Emperor energy, I think of one of the people who has filled a teacher
role in my life, Leesa Renée Hall. Leesa teaches anti-bias training particularly for em-
paths or highly sensitive introverted people,[*] but she has Emperor energy to me because her boundaries are solid, her leadership is defined and unquestionable, and she

---

[*]   At the time of writing this book, you can access Leesa's work and teachings via Patreon and on
Instagram @leesareneehall.

is level-headed in her work and steadfast in doing it (at least from my vantage point of student). All these very stable, practical traits represent Emperor energy.

Leesa's method of teaching is also through expressive writing for exploring biases. As you might have guessed, we all hold biases and beliefs about what pregnancy and birth must be because of how we were culturally conditioned to view pregnancy and birth. This makes freewriting or even simple word association an effective approach to beginning the important Emperor work of deciding the type of prenatal care you'll seek and building your birth plan. This way you are making decisions about your birth, not from an unexamined place of overculture thinking, but from a place that is truly aligned with your inner voice.

⤸ THE EMPEROR THEMES ⤸

planning, structure, thinking ahead, decisive, objective, detached, reparenting yourself, grounded, inflexible, giving, authority figure

EXERCISE

FREEWRITE TO UNEARTH YOUR SUBCONSCIOUS BIASES ABOUT BIRTH

While the Emperor can be your ally in the practical aspects of planning, your planning should also consider your feelings or cultural conditioning. Here is an exercise to help you start noticing the subconscious factors at play in your decision-making:

Without giving yourself time to overthink it, write down or say out loud what your mind associates with the following words:

- *Birth*
- *Pregnant*
- *Postpartum*
- *Breastfeeding/Bodyfeeding*

Then, without self-judgment, look at the ideas you associated with those words and make note of what you observe. Then maybe move into questioning whether it's in your best interest to keep those associations. For example, if the first word you associate with *postpartum* is *depression*, then that might be a conditioning worthy of your further examination and attention.

- When you imagine you and your future baby, where are you? Answer first quickly without taking too much time to think about it. Then follow it up with freewriting about the location where you think you'll birth. Please remember, don't judge yourself for what you're writing. It doesn't have to be shared with anyone, and it doesn't have to be perfectly fleshed out yet.

- Continuing to use freewriting, explore some limiting beliefs you may hold about how and where people in your culture birth. For example, do you think safe birth happens only outside the home in the medical-industrial complex? Do you think beautiful, spiritual births can happen only inside the home? Do you expect that birth is bigger than your body and you'll need medical assistance or pain medication? See what comes up and try to stay curious. Just keep writing.

- Write what you know, or don't know, about the following care providers: midwives (both CPM and CNM), obstetricians, doulas, nurses. Then after writing, research the different roles these different professionals play during birth.

- Write what you know, or don't know, about the following decisions you'll need to make during pregnancy and birth—feelings about testing and ultrasounds, pain management, continuous fetal monitoring versus intermittent monitoring, water birth, cervical exams, informed consent, eating and drinking during labor, medical induction of labor, use of IVs and antibiotics during labor, movement during labor, cascade of interventions, physiologic birth, Cesarean section surgical birth, and anything else that comes to mind. Write about these things, and then follow up by researching the evidence-based practices surrounding them and make your decisions for your own birth from an empowered place of your own research.

- Write what you know, or don't know, about the following decisions you'll need to make immediately after birth—delayed cord clamping or lotus birth, placenta encapsulation or smoothies, vaccinations, circumcision, skin-to-skin, keeping the baby on parents, the microbiome, bathing the baby, antibiotics, post-partum visitors/helpers, bodyfeeding, formula feeding, and anything else that comes to mind. Write what you know, share your opinions or biases, and then follow up with conducting your own evidence-based research.

Note that it is Emperor energy that often allows us to get through the less fun but necessary work we need to put toward bringing our plans to fruition. That might seem like a lot of homework I just listed, and since no amount of research or preparation ever guarantees anything ever, it can feel like, *Why bother putting in all this soul inquiry and knowledge acquisition?* You get out of this exercise what you put into it, even if that's simply the knowledge that you did your own due diligence.

The results of this exercise might be just the start of your birth plan. Don't expect a final product ready to print off and hand to your birth team at the end of this exercise. You don't necessarily have to come out of this exercise with all your decisions made, but examining the biases and expec-tations we hold around pregnancy, birth, and postpartum is an important first step in making decisions from an aligned place within, instead of sim-ply from a place of upholding the status quo.

Once you do feel like you are at a place to make some decisions, especially if you're choosing an out-of-home birth, you'll want to have a written version of your birth plan for the birth team to consult. The website Mamanatural .com has a great template with simple icons to indicate your choices to quickly and effectively communicate them to the team.

Note: When conducting self-led research to craft your birth plan, you can flip to "The Tens" chapter (page 105). These cards correlate to when birth happens, so this chapter includes information about the hormonal, physical, and environmental requirements of physiologic birth to bolster your understanding when making your birth choices.

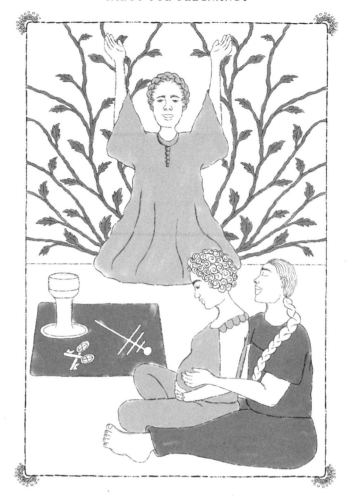

5–THE HIEROPHANT

"It's no secret that children often stimulate their parents to
reexamine or renew their religious beliefs. I believe that in
many cases this is a past life agreement between parent and
child to remind parents of their spiritual heritage."

—Walter Makichen, clairvoyant, *Spirit Babies:
How to Communicate with the Child You're Meant to Have*

You are already acting upon the energy of the Hierophant because you're reading
this book! This indicates to me that you're doing the work to learn something about
pregnancy, birth, and the spiritual, intuitive connection to those things.

If this card comes up in your spread, it's time to seek higher guidance from
someone who carries more wisdom on a subject than you. For the most part, my goal

with this book is to remind you of your own innate power—your intuition is smart, and you do have valid and valuable wisdom within your own body that is worthy of paying attention to, even though it doesn't come with a certificate or degree. But it is of course still a valuable thing to continue to learn from a place of being a curious student, both in the science of physiologic birth and in your spiritual practice.

This card could be telling you to take a birth class. Seek one that is not affiliated with the location where you plan to birth, so you know their information won't be biased toward catering to that particular birthing place or care provider. Or go ahead and take a birth class at the location affiliated with your birthplace but take another one somewhere else too. There are truly endless things to learn about birth; this field is a well that I have yet to fully tap myself and I've been insatiable about gaining more knowledge about birth for four solid and intentional years.

If taking a birth class is not accessible in your area or for your budget, then dive into the wealth of episodes on the podcast *Birthful* hosted by Adriana Lozada. It is chock-full of all the unbiased, evidence-based birth information you could want and also home to hundreds of birth stories. You might think that you just signed up to become a parent, not a birth worker, but becoming a student of pregnancy, birth, and postpartum will only work to your advantage, and it's what the Hierophant calls us to do.

This card could also be telling you to consult your hired birth professional(s) on whatever you're working through at the moment. Or it could be a sign to put in the time to read those pregnancy books you may be putting off. Or it could mean it's time to book a tarot or intuitive reading to gain clarity on your next moves.

❧ THE HIEROPHANT THEMES ❧

teacher, community, experts, guidance, wisdom, healer, religion, ritual

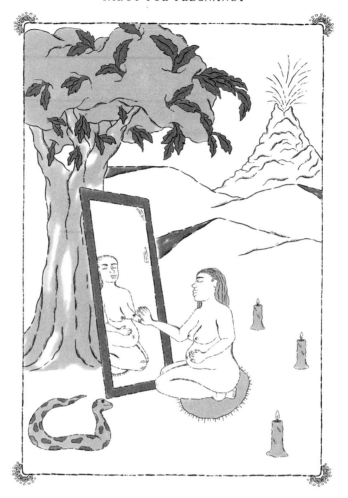

6–THE LOVERS

In the tarot, the Lovers could represent a choice that needs to be made, but note that there are no positive or negative attributes associated with this choice or the energy it presents. Punishment does not await you for making the "wrong" choice here. There is, indeed, no wrong choice, only the one you make and the lessons you learn.

If this card is not showing up in your spread as a choice, then it can be appearing to represent a balanced duality, partnership, or even a blissfulness. The Lovers embodies a balance between lunar and solar energies working in perfect tandem together.

In the Lovers, 1 + 1 doesn't just equal 2, it equals infinite potential. Each component, when combined, becomes greater than the sum of its individual parts when in aligned union.

Whether you find yourself in a partnership during your journey to pregnancy and parenthood or not, you can still tap into the joyful, balanced energy of this card within yourself or in relation to your baby.

⤳ THE LOVERS THEMES ⤶

balance, partnerships, duality, choices, connecting, bonding

EXERCISE

WRITE A LOVE LETTER

If this card comes to you or resonates with you during your fertility or pregnancy journey, I invite you to try this exercise.

Write a love letter to either yourself, your partner (either the one you have or the one you dream of having), or your baby (either born, conceived, fetal, or just an idea). You don't have to be an eloquent writer, and you don't even need to share this letter with another person if you don't want to. Authenticity and frankness matter more than your ability to conjure flowery phrases. Here are some suggestions for what to include in your letter to get you started:

- Something that makes you feel vulnerable to say/admit out loud
- How gorgeous/beautiful they/you are, then describe why
- How fulfilled you are by the life you have or will have together or by your whole self; how grateful you are to get to be living it with them/being you
- A lighthearted exclamation of the joy you feel in their presence/ when you're connecting to and spending time with yourself
- Say something corny or lovey-dovey to yourself, your partner (current or future), or your baby, something that makes the haters roll their eyes
- Name some parts of yourself that you feel are balanced or made better by their presence in your life, or if you're writing a letter to yourself, examine ways in which solar and lunar energies are beautifully and wholly balanced within you

If you choose to write a letter to the lover you want, not one that you currently have, I still suggest writing the letter in present tense—as if you already are experiencing, enjoying, and grateful for life with that person. For a simple spell, you can write your letter, fold the paper toward yourself three times, place the paper under a red or pink candle, and let the candle burn all the way down. You can dress or adorn the altar or candle with what-ever you'd like, such as fresh flowers, wine, chocolate, crystals, herbs (rose petals, passionflower, or juniper berries), to increase the potency of your spell. But what matters more than any fancy tool is your intention when writing your words or lighting the candle, truly believing that your vision is already on its way to you. Finish your letter with a prayer of gratitude for this person, as if it is already done. You can repeat this spell as often as you like.

If you wrote a letter to yourself, I suggest reading the letter aloud to yourself in the mirror, trying to make as much eye contact with yourself as possible. Soul-gazing can be an intense experience if you are not feeling a lot of love for your physical body, so feel free to take breaks if you need to, cry if you need to, but always finish off with returning to your own gaze at least briefly. Then I suggest placing the letter on your mirror where you get ready every day, or on your altar with some pink and red candles. If you wrote about a kind of love for yourself that you do not yet feel, you can do the same exact love-attracting spell detailed above but about yourself, not about a partner you're calling in.

If you wrote your letter to the partner you currently have, I suggest giv-ing it to them! Yes, even if you feel silly, awkward, or vulnerable—in fact, bonus points if you feel those discomforts but choose to put yourself out there anyway. Put it in an envelope tucked in with the regular mail, so they'll be surprised and see it without you needing to hand it to them directly.

If you wrote your letter to your future baby, I suggest putting it in their nursery, or wherever you're keeping the items you've prepared for them. If you're birthing in a hospital or birth center, put the letter in your packed bag. If you're birthing at home, put the letter in the room you think you'll likely give birth in. When you find it during labor it might just be the heart-ening boost to remind you of the love that brought you here, and the multi-plying love that is on the other side of birth.

If you wrote the letter to your current child, I suggest reading it to them like a children's book, regularly, so they can know the love that created them is infused all around them. Then put it in their baby book or the journal you keep for a delightful surprise for them to find later in life.

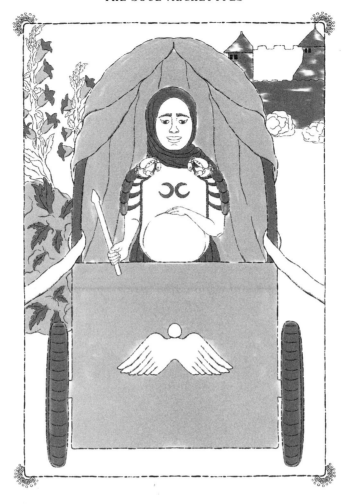

7–THE CHARIOT

"Keep some room in your heart for the unimaginable."
—Mary Oliver, queer poet and environmentalist

The Chariot comes into play when a care provider tells you that you'll have gestational diabetes because of your weight, or when a care provider warns that you'll be less likely to bodyfeed because of your skin color, or any of the myriad of ways people put you in a box. The Chariot is here to help you bust yourself out of that box and help you with the extra energy it will take to achieve that goal. This energy will assist you in putting in the work to get the outcome you want.

The Chariot is associated with the astrological sign of Cancer, which is represented by the crab, and the nuance to the energy of the Chariot can't be fully fleshed out without talking about the crab. One of the ways the Chariot helps us barrel ahead on our goals is with the shell—protecting our softness and our vulnerabilities until we get where we need to be, where it's safe to shed our shell. So be cautioned against staying in Chariot mode too long so you don't stay hardened or spend too much time in a safe-feeling shell that you've long since outgrown.

Hold this truth with you as you embark on the goal of obtaining the care and the birth you deserve. You are deserving of compassionate, individualized, trauma-informed, unbiased, accessible care. It is your birthright. You have the right to seek that goal until you find it, and you have the right to change your mind, too, if your birthplace or care provider proves to be incompetent with providing you with these things. A safe, respectful, un-traumatizing, empowering, and birthing parent–led birth is a human right, not a luxury.

Likewise, allow your view of "safety" to evolve. Stepping out of an old mode of being for a time does make you vulnerable, but take heart in knowing that your old chariot wasn't as safe as it seemed anyway, and you can build an even better idea of safety with what you know now and what you're learning.

❧ THE CHARIOT THEMES ☙

making progress, drive, moving forward, momentum, determination,
not taking no for an answer, shedding an old shell that doesn't fit anymore

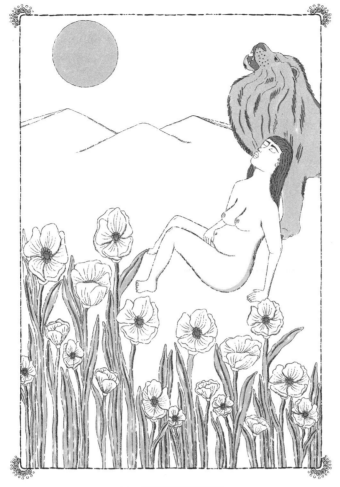

8–STRENGTH

The energy of the Strength card is an immense teacher in pregnancy and birth because its power doesn't lie in an outward expression of force or will. It is in the calm reserve. It is the softening and expanding of the body to accommodate a fetus and birth a baby. This is Strength and it has nothing to prove.

When this card comes up in a reading about pregnancy or birth, it might mean *do nothing* or at the very least *wait and see.* If you don't know where you stand about a decision, a test, a procedure, and the like, ask if it can wait (it almost always can) and then wait for clarity to reveal itself at the unrushed pace of your intuitive knowing. The restraint required to pause before acting requires an immense amount of self-control and strength. But since that muscle doesn't visibly show, we often don't give due credit to the power available to us in this energy.

It's probably obvious that this makes it a rather mature energy, so when you feel yourself slipping into ego-only-driven or reactionary tendencies or giving into pressure even though your intuition is requesting you do otherwise, call back your power and remember who you are. (I use the verbiage of ego-*only*-driven because of course ego is at the table. It's present in all of us; I just mean that it shouldn't be the sole voice from which we make decisions.)

You can receive input without reacting. You can trust yourself to act and decide appropriately when the time is right to do so.

As pertains to birth specifically, we can look at the fact that childbirth is one of the most extreme displays of athleticism and endurance the human body can perform. From toweling a sweat-beaded brow to offering birthing people sips of water before their next contraction, the parallels are obvious. Endurance is required, and we don't know exactly when it will end, but we will be allowed to rest at last.

And yet, true to the meaning of the Strength card, the only way through this high-endurance extreme sport known as birth is to become utterly soft, to surrender to the intensity. And it takes so much more work and strength than we ever expect to do *less* in birth.

The Strength card is also bound up with our sexuality, which may seem out of place if you were reading any other tarot guide, but because this particular tarot guide is talking about pregnancy and birth, it should make all the sense in the world. The act of sex with ourselves or with a partner teaches us the physical manifestation of letting go of the edge we cling to in order to float down the stream of ecstasy.

You know how when you "try" really hard to have an orgasm, it suddenly seems impossible? This is what I mean when I say the Strength card's power is in letting go. Ultimately, we tap into our greatest power through release, whether you're releasing through crowning or through orgasm.

⦃ STRENGTH THEMES ⦄
restraint, resolve, inner power, calm, sexuality, pausing before acting, subtle power, courage, perseverance, strength is softness, creative power

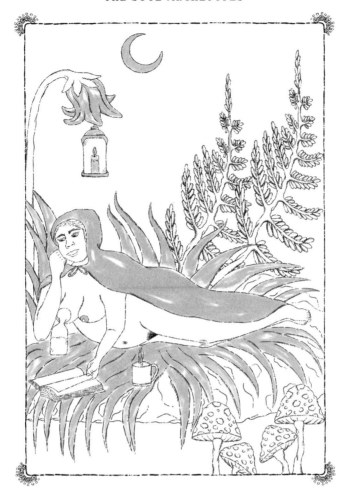

9–THE HERMIT

"Listen to yourself and in that quietude you might hear the voice of God."

—Maya Angelou, mother, poet, and civil rights activist

The Hermit is often a call to withdraw from the outer world. For some folks, the entirety of their pregnancy will ask this of them. Others might only feel this call near the end of their pregnancy or during postpartum. This pull to explore inward is of course necessary for pregnancy, but it particularly resonates for postpartum.

White-supremacist, colonial, patriarchal, capitalist, ableist American culture, as it is right now at least, doesn't have a whole lot of ritual around the postpartum period. We're culturally disconnected from our sacred postpartum practices that once honored the open channel that we are during postpartum and tended to our healing slowly and intentionally. Now, we go out and about with our newborns, we don't honor rest, and we don't honor our body's call to retreat and withdraw from the world. We often pick up and go on about life as if nothing even happened. Capitalism forces us to go back to work sooner than is tenable for the requirements of healing. We attempt to "get our body back," we don't ask for help, we socialize instead of taking a nap. Society supports and cosigns this unsustainable way of being postpartum, expecting the most of us and punishing us if we refuse.

The Hermit reminds us to fuck all that noise. You do not owe anyone access to yourself or your baby postpartum. Stay home if you can. Stay in if you can. Go as slow as you can. There is no rush to figure out your new normal. Your lochia* is there to act as the barometer for whether you're doing too much (because you'll bleed heavier if you're not honoring your need for rest). Your milk comes in easier, and stays flowing more regularly at home, too, when you are in the comfort of your own space.

If you do decide to offer people the privilege of entering the microbiome of your home, then make sure they know the space they'll be asked to respect and protect during the sacred recovery period that is postpartum. I advise against visitors; instead make it known that only helpers are welcome in your postpartum space, folks who are comfortable coming in and doing what chores need to be done, bringing you food, or looking after your newborn or older children long enough for you to nap or shower. Anyone who will expect you to host them, who will hold your baby too long and not pay attention to their rooting,† or who doesn't respect the boundaries you've set for yourself or your baby is going to have to wait to visit after you've healed and gotten your footing.

It should be noted that it is capitalist white supremacy culture that makes us feel like we should be doing the most postpartum. It didn't used to be this way, and for many other cultures that are still rooted in their Indigenous traditions, it's not this way. So if the Hermit is revealing itself to you, one way you could go inward is by researching your ancestral cultural practices and traditions around the postpartum time.

If colonialism has severed access to your ancestry, or you simply don't know what to research or where to start, the Hermit is also a great ally in meditation. And

....

* Lochia (pronounced *la-kee-uh*) is the bleeding that persists after birth, beginning heavy and bright red, and slowly fading over the course of your first several weeks postpartum.

† Rooting is a reflex where babies open their mouths and "root" around looking for a nipple and is a signal of hunger in infants.

the question of what your ancestral practices around postpartum are and were is absolutely a question you can meditate on to uncover them within yourself. Use your meditation to call in and ask your ancestors for guidance. Your cells and your ancestors remember the answer.

☽ THE HERMIT THEMES ☾

inward reflection, inner journey, antisocial, introversion, solitude, meditation, connecting with the human you're growing, disengagement with the outer world

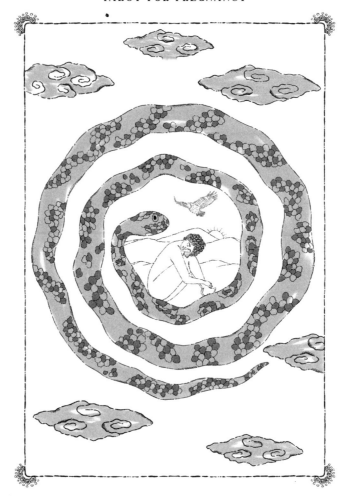

10–THE WHEEL OF FORTUNE

In the Wheel of Fortune, we find ourselves face-to-face with familiar themes in our lives and maybe thinking, *I thought I was over this. Didn't I heal this already?* Healing is not linear, it spirals in on itself, but fortunately, each time a familiar theme comes up again, that usually means we are spiraling closer to the center of it. But this nonlinear healing means that eventually we can all expect to revisit something we thought we were over or out of, especially when we are on the enormously transformative and reality-shattering journey that is the path to and in parenthood.

When the Wheel comes to us, we are being gifted an opportunity to revisit that familiar theme in our lives and see what new tools we might have in our toolbox to address the issue. If we choose to ignore what's begging to be revisited, begging to be healed, that's okay, it will almost certainly come up again, and likely be louder, more insistent, and even less comfortable than before.

This archetype has about a million possible variations because how the Wheel will show up in our lives will be as unique as each of our individual life experiences. So I'm going to use one imaginary example, and then you might be able to start to consider what this archetype has to offer you on your parenthood journey.

Imagine: In childhood you experienced some trauma with adults who exercised their power of authority over you excessively, and indiscriminately, subsequently inhibiting the growth of your sense of autonomy over your life or control over your body. This trauma caused your childhood and adolescent self to have an excessive fear of authority figures, which showed up in silent panic attacks that looked like shutting down, maybe in class with a teacher who wasn't sensitive to your needs, or at the doctor's office, and so on. This manifested in avoiding ever going to the doctor in early adulthood, even when needed, because there was a fear that your past trauma would inhibit you from being able to speak up for yourself or your needs, as you still felt intimidated by authority figures.

Fast-forward: You are now a pregnant person, and you have your first appointment with the doctor you're interviewing to see if you'd like to continue with their care throughout the rest of your pregnancy and for your birth. During this appointment, the mannerisms and air of this doctor are triggering the memories you have of childhood trauma from unchecked authority figures. You have now spiraled back around on the Wheel of Fortune and find yourself experiencing feelings you haven't felt since adolescence, feeling like you don't have a choice about whether you go to this doctor, feeling like you have to do what they say without question, feeling yourself clam up and become afraid to ask your valid questions because the adults in your childhood made you feel like your questions and concerns were irrelevant.

You have a choice here. You could take the gift that the Wheel of Fortune is offering, do whatever therapy, meditation, healing work, or the like that you need in order to learn how to let your inner child speak up in the face of intimidating authority. Then, you can bring a support person or your partner with you to your next appointment, utilize the new tools in your toolbox, and let this doctor who triggers you know that you will be seeking care from another professional.

Or you could refuse the gift that the Wheel of Fortune is trying to offer. You could deny your inner voice who is begging you to be heard, and you could placate yourself with a blanket like, *What do I know? The doctor knows best.*

You continue attending your prenatal visits and this doctor has given you dietary suggestions that are out of alignment with your usual diet, foods that typically make you feel good every day, but you heed their orders despite the negative changes in how your body feels. You express interest in movement during labor, delayed cord clamping, bodyfeeding, and your doctor replies with, "Well, we'll see how it goes," implying an expectation that things will go wrong, implying that they have no intention of doing everything in their power to assist your birth in going in alignment with your wishes.

Fast-forward to your birth: Even though nothing is wrong, and you are moving through and with your surges just fine, you are hooked up to a continuous fetal monitor and therefore confined to your bed. We are at a familiar point on the Wheel of Fortune again, and again, you have an opportunity to do things differently, spiraling closer on your Wheel toward your truth.

Again, you have a choice: You can pull up your research on the efficacy of intermittent fetal monitoring and its safety for low-risk births and the evidence that continuous fetal monitoring has been proven to cause an increase in unnecessary interventions, and ask to be taken off the monitor. Or you simply move your body the way you need to regardless, and your movement knocks the monitor out of place and a nurse has to come in and fix it, but so what? You're finally starting to realize that everyone there, the doctor, the nurses, were all hired *by* you to work *for* you, and the previously seemingly insurmountable weight of their authority starts to shrink as you begin to recognize and claim your own power and authority in the space.

Or you could refuse the gift that the Wheel of Fortune is trying to give you again; you could remain in bed, trying not to move so that the monitor doesn't get bumped off, so you don't have to bother the nurses. Your surges are even more unbearable on your back confined to the bed, and a nurse frequently comes in to remind you that you can have an epidural at any time. She keeps repeating, "There's no medal for giving birth without an epidural," which makes you feel small, patronized, and foolish for having your own hopes, dreams, and goals for your own birth. Despite the fact that your surges were more bearable when you were walking around, or swaying your hips with your birth partner before you got the hospital, you still feel capable of dealing with the surges you're experiencing in the bed, and don't feel like you need or want an epidural, but you're getting the strong vibe that the nurse is annoyed with your stated birth preferences, and like maybe she wants you to get an epidural so that you're an easier patient for her to attend to.

She has lots of other patients to attend to on the floor that night, and you don't want to be a bother. You relent to getting the epidural, so you are less loud and less needy. You notice your surges slow down and start to space apart now that the epi-dural has kicked in. The nurses and doctor notice, too, so they administer Pitocin to "move things along," and since they didn't even ask for consent this time, you don't even have the opportunity to protest, even though you read about Pitocin and it's on your birth preferences not to use it. The familiar feeling surfaces that your body and your choices are not in your hands.

Fast-forward to postpartum: You're sent home from the hospital. No doctors, no nurses. You wonder, *If they knew better all along to the point where they made all their choices for you, then how can you go home with this baby and be trusted with them alone?*

Because of the drugs you were on during birth, your milk is slow to come in, and when it does, the stress and anxiety you're feeling makes your supply low, making you have a never-satiated baby. Your disempowering experience in birth is leaking into your vulnerable postpartum time in the form of feeling unequipped to care for your baby, or as though your baby isn't safe with you or the decisions you're making on their behalf.

Instead of educating you on the normal supply and demand required of early lactation in order for your milk to come in, your pediatrician instead goes with what they know, what they can measure, and suggests supplementing with formula until your supply increases. But you, knowing the physiology of bodyfeeding, know that it's a supply-and-demand circuit, and you know that supplementing without a plan to increase your own supply will do nothing but decrease your own supply.

Again, the Wheel of Fortune has brought you back to a familiar theme. An author-ity figure is giving you information that contradicts what you know to be true about physiology and about your own body. The adrenaline of the doctor's visit alone is dry-ing you right up. But again, the Wheel of Fortune gives you a choice: You could re-spectfully disagree with your pediatrician and seek out a lactation consultant who is trained in the normal physiology of a newborn bodyfeeding relationship to help get you on track in a way that takes care of you and your baby. Or you could go against your better judgment and against your own choices and supplement with the formula sam-ples. But because the pediatrician didn't give you a plan of how to get your own supply up or a referral for a lactation consultant or a support group, your own milk supply begins to shrink and is all but gone within the first three months of your baby's life.

While this story is fictional and not about any one parent, it is a common tale. After reading the story, you might now be able to imagine the fictional parent's trajectory

through parenthood and the ways in which their unhealed relationship with authority figures will continue to show up in their parenting. Maybe their child will have a
hard time seeing them as an authority figure or respecting them. Or maybe they will
reenact the same excessive and indiscriminate use of authority and unchecked
power as an unhealthy expression of their own unhealed childhood trauma. Either
way, it is unavoidably true that until addressed head-on (and likely more than once),
this issue is going to continue showing up in that person's life.

This might make the Wheel of Fortune feel awful, scary, and rather depressing,
but it's not! It comes up only as an opportunity to break the cycles in which we keep
ourselves and to learn to do better by ourselves and by our children. (See "The
World," page 239, for further exploration). It often shows up as a means of reclaiming our personal power.

❧ THE WHEEL OF FORTUNE THEMES ☙

*old patterns, spiraling inward, unexamined wounds, taking a chance, cycles,
rebirth, familiar themes, inner child*

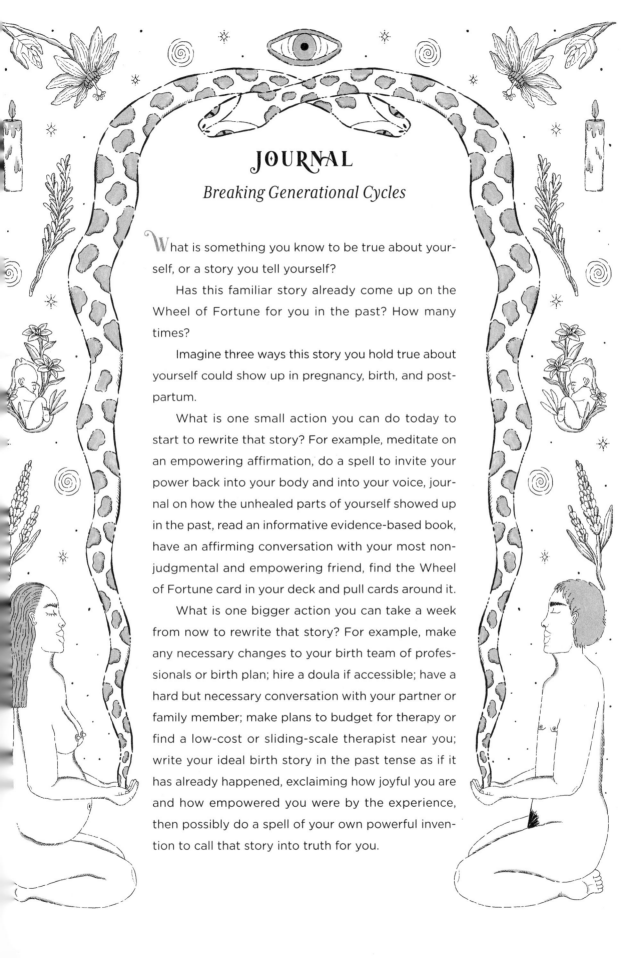

JOURNAL

Breaking Generational Cycles

What is something you know to be true about yourself, or a story you tell yourself?

Has this familiar story already come up on the Wheel of Fortune for you in the past? How many times?

Imagine three ways this story you hold true about yourself could show up in pregnancy, birth, and postpartum.

What is one small action you can do today to start to rewrite that story? For example, meditate on an empowering affirmation, do a spell to invite your power back into your body and into your voice, journal on how the unhealed parts of yourself showed up in the past, read an informative evidence-based book, have an affirming conversation with your most nonjudgmental and empowering friend, find the Wheel of Fortune card in your deck and pull cards around it.

What is one bigger action you can take a week from now to rewrite that story? For example, make any necessary changes to your birth team of professionals or birth plan; hire a doula if accessible; have a hard but necessary conversation with your partner or family member; make plans to budget for therapy or find a low-cost or sliding-scale therapist near you; write your ideal birth story in the past tense as if it has already happened, exclaiming how joyful you are and how empowered you were by the experience, then possibly do a spell of your own powerful invention to call that story into truth for you.

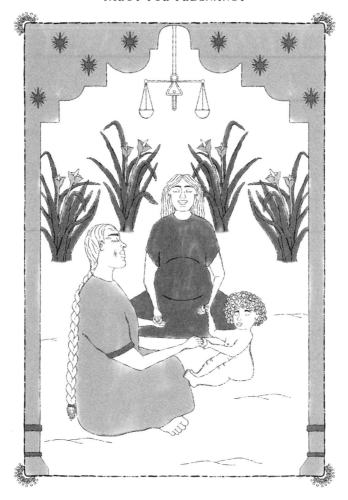

11–JUSTICE

"Does the justice you advocate for publicly mirror the justice you practice privately? Do the rules you live by to navigate the external world align with your internal code of ethics?"

—Sarah T. Cargill, artist, cultural worker,
and spiritual care practitioner*

Justice is a call to action to utilize your parenthood path to get more in alignment with your ethics and live them daily. While we are all going to become ancestors one day, regardless of whether we procreate or not, the choice to continue your family

....

* Sarah is also the host of the podcast *Tarot for the End of Times* and founder and owner of Snakeskin Tarot. Find her online at www.sarahtcargill.com and www.snakeskintarot.com.

tree is the choice to one day become somebody's direct elder. Is the family lineage you're a part of something you want to perpetuate?

Values-driven pregnancy and parenting goes beyond teaching our kids to "be kind."

If you are a person who holds white privilege, class privilege, or any other kind of privilege that has increased your likelihood of thriving in this world, you have the opportunity to use your journey to and in parenthood as an opportunity to become antiracist so that you do not continue to pass on the dangerous legacy of white supremacy to your lineage.*

I am not an antiracism educator, nor would it be appropriate for me to be one given my lived experience, but this book would be missing a piece of the parenting puzzle if I skipped over talking about pregnancy and parenthood as an opportunity for generational healing and dismantling white supremacy.

I've learned through my own inner work that dismantling white supremacy cannot be a passive endeavor, and that I must be devoted to prioritizing the lives and safety of BIPOC children over the innocence of my own white-passing child. I've learned (and keep learning over and over again) that it doesn't matter what I say to my child, he's paying more attention to what I do. So that's why for any white folks reading this book, the inner work is a step that cannot be skipped, because we can't teach something we don't embody.

For some of us, gentle, respectful parenting is going to be a means of breaking generational trauma. For parents who are descendants of enslaved people, body-feeding can be a form of generational healing.† For some of us, prioritizing joy and letting our children be messy and curious will help reparent our inner child. No matter what it is, healing is a political act that will impact the next generation that you're birthing and raising up, and this is how for the parenthood path, healing is an act of Justice.

---

* In the resource list on page 158 you will find books and educators to guide you on your antiracism journey.

† Once again, I recommend the book *The Big Letdown* by Kimberly Seals Allers for a whole education on how the history of wet-nursing during chattel slavery still impacts bodyfeeding attitudes today, as well as how health care providers' racist bias, and predatory formula companies targeting the Black community, all work against Black birthing people in their bodyfeeding journeys.

Justice might also be enacted (in part) by cloth diapering, bodyfeeding, second-hand baby items, baby-led weaning instead of buying packaged baby foods—all things that are more environmentally sustainable choices.[*]

Even simply looking at children as individuals who are human—and parenting them from that place—is revolutionary compared to the way many of us were raised. There are many ways to begin choosing a new path: electing a home birth if that's accessible and makes sense for you, working toward normalizing a shift back to a way of birthing before it was erased by colonization, and funding Black and Indigenous midwives.

There is so much work to be done, internal and external, to dismantle the devastating legacy of capitalism, of white supremacy, of the patriarchy, and colonialism, and every one of us has something to contribute and a call to answer (see also "Judgment," page 236).

∻ JUSTICE THEMES ⧫

doing the right thing even if it's the hard thing, balance, integrity,
living from your ethics, trusting your own discernment

---

[*] Also, always acknowledging that environmental justice is about so much more than individual personal choices toward sustainability and more about dismantling the extractive practices of imperial, capitalist white supremacy. The world's wealthiest 1 percent is responsible for CO_2 emissions double that of populations driven into poverty by capitalism. Humanity is not inherently extractive and taxing on the Earth, but the colonial Eurocentric way of living a "civilized" life definitely is.

TAROT SPREAD FOR FURTHERING JUSTICE THROUGH PARENTING

Here is a suggested tarot spread to explore how you specifically are called to further justice in the world through your parenting path. Do this spread as many times as you need to during pregnancy and throughout your life as a parent, because the work is never over:

Find the Justice card in your deck, and place it at the center of the spread.

Below: What do I need to see in order to show up for Justice in my journey to and in parenthood?

Behind: What in my past or family legacy needs to be healed for future generations?

Above: What guiding principle will lead me in my pursuit of Justice?

Ahead: How can I show up for Justice moving forward?

You can keep pulling more cards off those four points to further elaborate and deepen the conversation.

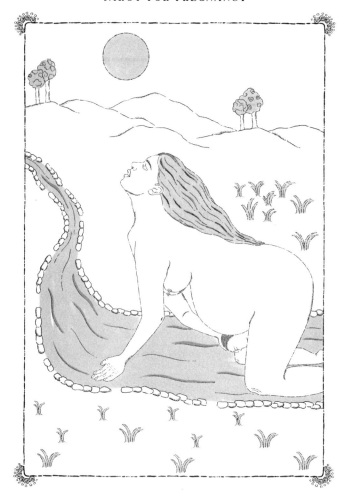

12–THE HANGED ONE

"Transformation is often more about unlearning than learning."

—Richard Rohr

We were taught through culture, media, and patriarchal messaging to believe that birth is a dramatic, screaming, painful endeavor. This punitive idea dates back to the idea of the original sin and the idea that the pain of childbirth was a form of punishment.

We can reject this falsehood by noticing birth's beauty, birth as an opportunity for transcendence and divinity, birth's ebbs and flows or even its possibility for orgasmic elation, instead of responding to the patriarchal notion of pain as punishment with the idea that pain could also be avoided.*

This is why, when we're preparing for our birth, we need to unlearn this messaging just as much as we need to learn about physiologic birth itself. This stripping down and spiraling back inward toward the truth is Hanged One energy.

The Hanged One is the ultimate surrender, and pregnancy is a major teacher for the energy this card asks us to embody. Surrendering and letting go are some of the biggest lessons of pregnancy that get driven home most potently during labor and birth.

Whether it's pregnancy symptoms calling us to adjust to the slow pace of postpartum or pairing down the mental and physical clutter in our lives to make space for what is to come, the Hanged One is the bittersweet of letting go.

This hearkens to the leap of the Fool but with intention and awareness instead of naïveté. The Hanged One speaks deeply to the liminal space that is the final weeks of pregnancy when you must surrender into the mystery of knowing when your baby is going to come. This is the energy that comes through when it's time to release our babies to the world. This card is the actual work of moving through a transition and bringing something to its conclusion.

The lesson is that it's safe to wait. Suspension is not a bad thing, our on-to-the-next-thing culture is just averse to the deep (and often uncomfortable) magic available in liminal spaces. It's safe to let go. It's safe to release control.

⊰ THE HANGED ONE THEMES ⊱

suspension, surrender, letting go, trust fall, different perspective from a new angle, transformation, breakthrough, unlearning, shaking habits

....

* The (largely white women–led) feminist response to that patriarchal messaging was the epidural—a way to opt out of the sensations of childbirth.

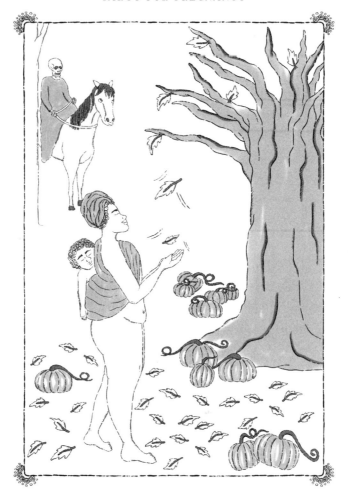

13–DEATH

My mother spent the first couple decades of her nursing career as a labor and delivery nurse, and then the last couple decades of her career as a hospice nurse. She was an L&D nurse in the 1970s and '80s before rooming in was standard practice, so while all the other nurses would let the newborns cry it out in the nursery, my mom would neglect her other duties to hold and soothe the babies that should have been with their parents.

Years later, in hospice work (which is end-of-life care), she was the one all the other hospice nurses would call in when it was "time." They were uncomfortable being there when someone died, but she wasn't. She of course wouldn't have called it by this title at the time, but I know her to be a death doula. If the patient had family with them, she would explain to the family everything that was going to happen as their loved one transitioned, say a prayer with them, and support them through it. If the patient had no family there, she would make sure she was present when they passed, singing that Sarah McLachlan song, "Angel," as they went.*

She didn't do this because she was indifferent to, unmoved by, or unaffected by death. Knowing my mother, she was crying her way through it every single time and would likely be deeply affected by the loss of one of her patients for the rest of the week. Just as she respected the babies who needed accompaniment when they are new to this world, she respected that elders also need accompaniment on their way out. She did this because she had a respect for the transition that death is, not something to be feared and avoided, but tended to and supported, just like birth.

In this way, we can culturally draw a parallel between death and birth. We're willing to come witness it after the event has happened (in the form of a funeral or visiting to see the baby) but witnessing the spiritual transition into or out of a body makes us uncomfortable.

When I was younger, I always found it odd how my mom could go from one end of the spectrum to the other, seeing people on their way into this world and then seeing them on their way out. But this was because I was assigning an inherent "good" to birth and an inherent "bad" to death, instead of seeing them for what they are—two equal sides of the same coin.

The Death card is one of the major reasons I wanted to write this book. Because even though the energy of the Death card has truly *so* much to do with the transitions we go through during birth, and the milestones we and our children pass through during parenthood, it can make parents fearful of consulting the tarot about their pregnancy or children at all, for fear that when this card comes up, it's indicative of a literal loss of life. I suppose it can mean that, but frankly, so can lots of other cards that talk about letting go and transitioning. The bodily functions of death and birth hold equal weight, so I don't think the enormity of physical, bodily death with all its nuance can be relegated to one card. There could be a whole book on tarot for death, as this is just as big of a life event as birth. So, in this chapter, I'm referring to the energy of the Death card as it pertains to birth and parenthood.

It's also a good time to note that tarot readings, for pregnancy in particular but really in all situations, are more about gaining clarity in the moment than

....

* My mom would tell me stories about birds that would appear in the windows after they went that she knew intuitively was their spirit leaving their body, and to this day I consider certain birds to be transitioned folks. I was raised staunchly Christian, and my mom still considers herself thus, but it's in these small ways that the pagan, Earth-based spirituality and belief in animism lives on covertly in my lineage.

necessarily divining the future. The future is not a fixed thing; we have influence over how things go depending on the choices we make and the choices other people make.

The energy of the Death archetype is one of an inevitable transition. The Hanged One is where we did all the work of surrendering and letting go, and in Death, it's already done, inevitable. It's the umbilical cord falling off when the time is right after your baby arrives—it happens in its own time and can't be rushed. If the Hanged One is pregnancy or the final weeks of waiting for your baby to come (all the work you put in to surrender to becoming a parent), then Death is birth (the final release after complete surrender).

I can assure you that Death card energy will come at the time of your birth, and this is the death of your old self. Who you were as a pregnant person is gone. Life as you know it will be utterly altered forever with no going back. And maybe now that I put it like that, you can see that there is indeed something to grieve. For a first-time parent, losing who you were before you were a parent is a huge transition that will feel like a very real loss. You might even grieve the loss of having your partner all to yourself. You might grieve the loss of having your body all to yourself if you are bodyfeeding your newborn. If this isn't your first child, the loss of that uninterrupted and unshared bond you have with your firstborn will be something to mourn too.

It's okay to give yourself space to grieve these losses, and here acceptance is key. Not because those losses aren't real, and not that they should be minimized, but fighting against the reality of those losses and denying yourself your right and space to grieve almost certainly can cause extra unnecessary strife. You don't need to keep reaching back for a version of your life that is no longer possible with the addition of this new human. You don't need to expect yourself to be capable of everything you previously could get done in one day. You don't need to keep your grip on relationships that prove to be too taxing, unsupportive, or unnourishing to this brand-new version of you.

Death card energy wants you to sit with what *is* instead of wishing for something that can no longer be. After all, a birth and a rebirth happened, too (or is about to happen), which requires the slow work of building and rebuilding from scratch. Learning a new normal is in order now.

◁ DEATH THEMES ▷

endings, seasons turning, inevitable shifts, transition, freedom,
release, rebirth, autumn

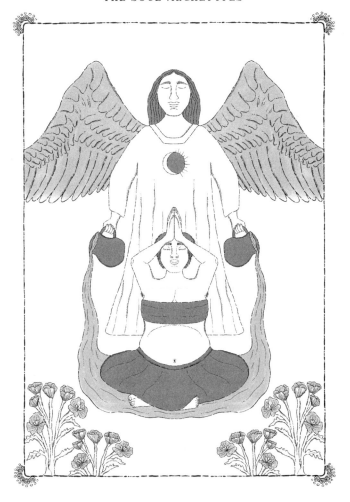

14-TEMPERANCE

"It is important to have a good relationship with the warriors (ancestors) because they teach us the difference between caution and cowardice, between courage and foolhardiness. They protect us both by steering us away from danger and by providing a feeling of confidence when a perilous situation must be faced."

—Yeye Luisah Teish, high priestess, artist, and author[*]

....

[*] Yeye Luisah Teish is an Iyanifa and Oshun chief in Yoruba tradition. She is celebrated internationally in Goddess circles as a writer and ritual-maker, and is the author of the globally celebrated classic spiritual text *Jambalaya: A Natural Woman's Book of Personal Charms and Practical Rituals*.

Temperance almost always shows up as a disembodied, nonhuman energy (at least not currently embodied or currently human). It might not even be an energy that we are aware of because it's acting on our behalf without our awareness, beyond the veil. It can be hard for us to even fathom Temperance, as this is not a humanly attainable level of understanding and grace.

When we are pregnant, it has been divinely cosigned for us to continue our ancestral line, so our ancestors and angels are heavily present with us during this time. You might find yourself feeling more ethereal, more connected to universal consciousness when you're pregnant, and this consistent, protective presence of your ancestors, spirit guides, and angels is just one of the reasons for that.

When this card shows up, it might be asking you to seek that center, even if getting there and staying there is unrealistic for humans. Whether you're pregnant or postpartum, weed out any extremes in your daily life, and make a practice of routinely coming back to your center through meditation, prayer, connection to the earth, or even just moments of quiet without any stimuli.

In birth, and often during pregnancy and parenthood, Temperance shows up as your divine protector. Moments like birth are when our angels, guides, and ancestors truly come through and protect us. You don't necessarily need to call upon them for this to happen, but if it comforts you to do so, then by all means, talk to them, invite them in, and don't forget how divinely protected you are.

You are protected and held. When you have no one else in the material world, you have *them*. Know this untouchable truth and hold it in your heart—expect the best for yourself. Expect protection, expect luck, expect good things to befall you.

For Black birthing folks in particular, expecting a good, positive birth experience might feel impractical and unrealistic given the white-supremacist cards stacked against you, influencing the statistics you've heard too many times. One of my mentors in my birthwork journey who I consider to embody this angel energy is the founder of Ancient Song Doula Services, Chanel Porchia-Albert. As she says, "We inherited a lot of ancestral trauma, yes, but we also inherited a lot of ancestral hope. We wouldn't be here without ancestral hope."

It's that exact ancestral hope that will be guiding and protecting you during birth. You can depend on that.

❧ TEMPERANCE THEMES ❦
angels, spirit guides, ancestors, divine protection, balanced duality, patience

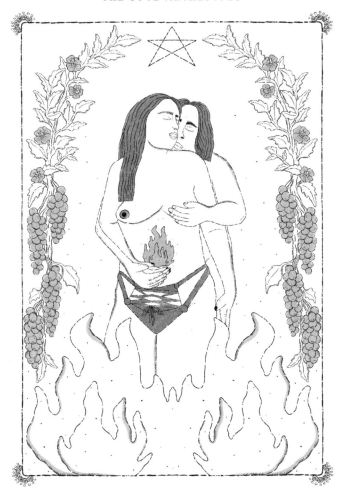

15–THE DEVIL

While my interpretation is not the common reading of the Devil archetype, in pregnancy and parenthood, I believe the Devil card shows up as an opportunity to re-examine our learned shame, or anything that keeps us from being free. These parts of us, when unexamined or unresolved, could manifest as fear, guilt, addiction, sexual suppression, negative self-talk, low expectations for our body's capabilities in birth, body shame, or an imbalanced relationship with bodily autonomy, not to mention any other number of ways we suppress our identities.

Under the white-supremacist purity-culture patriarchy, there are about a billion ways that we've been conditioned to accept and expect a punitive response if we ever question the societally accepted rules, challenge them, or further dare to discard them and unabashedly do our own thing. As a result, it makes all the sense in the world that we would try to keep ourselves small or come off as "modest." On a cellular level, this is the way of being that we've learned will keep us safe, because inhabiting our wholeness has historically made us a target.

If this card surfaces for you, and your query was related to your pregnancy, birth, or any other part of the spectrum of your sexuality, you are being called to do some shadow work and get curious about whether you truly benefit from the chains that bind you (that is, the rules we unquestioningly follow).

In my opinion, the traditional patriarchal, puritanical read on the Devil card is to beware of this archetype as a trap, as if it is out to get us and tempt us into evildoing or overindulgence. This archetype is merely pointing to the trap in which we've already agreed to keep ourselves, whether it was initially put there by society, past traumas, or any other negative experiences where we learned to hide or withhold.

When this card comes up, it's good to ask, *Do I really need to be this small and self-conscious? Do I really need to feel so guilty about XYZ?* (*XYZ* usually refers to the other cards surrounding it in the spread.) *What are some ways I'm restraining myself when I'm really longing to be free?* And so on.

Many will become pregnant via the act of sexual intercourse. Some might find newfound sexual revelry in their pregnant body. Feeling even less willing to exhibit sexual freedom once their body is hosting a fetus is also common. The act of birth is the culmination of the body's reproductive journey. When we allow ourselves to feel birth, it is by definition a sexual act. Birth requires feeling safe with who is in the room, produces the same hormones that our body produces during sex, eventually requires a huge release and letting go, and requires a mentally focused state of mind. All these similarities to sex remain true regardless of whether we personally want to look at birth as sexual.

If we are holding a blockage in our sexual expression or sexual freedom, that will likely try to reveal itself during birth and halt the enormous expansion and transformation that is transition. This can show up in those moments where our bodies are asking us to let go of modesty, but we want to stay covered up even if our skin is sensitive and uncomfortable and demands freedom from a bra. This can show up when our bodies require that we go inward to tap into a primal brainwave, but our thinking brain is afraid to release control, keeping us too conscious of everything and everyone else around us. And this can show up when our bodies are asking us to let go to release our babies, but we can't surrender and relax our pelvic floor because we are ashamed of the possibility of defecation.

The Devil card is a beautiful invitation to start doing the intense shadow work of dismantling how the Devil itself shows up in your life, preferably before or during, so you can start to work on, or at least notice and be aware of, the ways in which this archetype might be restricting you during labor. Some modality of therapy, or if therapy is inaccessible, at the very least a consultation with your least judgmental, sex-positive friend might help you start to shed the layers of shame that will do you no favors in pregnancy or birth.

It should also be noted that if this card is showing up in your spread as representative of someone else in your life, it is indicative that they are acting from a place of their wounding and their unexamined ego space. They're in their trap, and they want you in it with them. These people can be harmless until something happens, and then they're usually not so harmless anymore. In fact, they have the potential to cause immense amounts of harm. The common phrase *hurt people hurt people* comes to mind. But we can't force anyone else to go inward and look at their own shadows, so it's best to keep a safe distance from these folks while you are trying to preserve a certain state of mind during pregnancy, and definitely do not invite them to be involved in your birth in any capacity.

⊰ THE DEVIL THEMES ⊱

shame around sexuality, bondage, ego, self-doubt, imbalance, lack of clarity, the harm of purity culture, an opportunity for healing, invitation into freedom

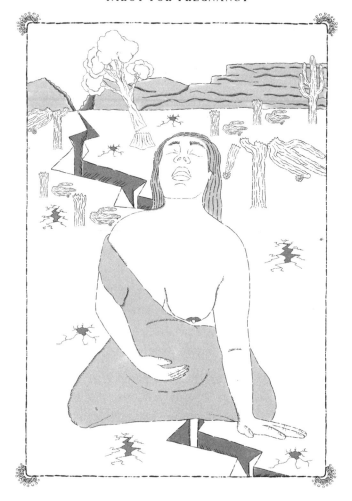

16–THE TOWER

The Tower is an intense, immense, but healthy burn that allows new growth to come through after the destruction. At the time of my writing, we are still in a global pandemic, uprisings have occurred calling for the United States to reckon with its violent, dehumanizing, racist, colonial legacy, and we're only at the beginning. The revolution is well under way. The brutality and disregard for Black people has been horrific, which necessitated an ongoing uprising and ultimately makes any equivalent destruction necessary. This is quintessential Tower energy. It's ugly, and it wakes us the fuck up. It's a privilege to be writing this book at this time, as a part of my contribution to fuel the flames.

While the Tower can manifest in a lot of ways in our lives, I think of the intensity of sensations we feel during labor. The intensity is on purpose. We go into labor as a previous self, and we come out of it utterly leveled, humbled, and ready to write a new fresh story, one where we are the parent. So, I'm going to utilize this chapter to talk about the sensations of labor and birth and how to cope through the storm that is the Tower.

Our perceptions influence our sensations, in the same way that a Pepsi Clear doesn't quite taste like Pepsi because it isn't meeting our visual expectations of what Pepsi tastes like. And it's little wonder that our perceptions of the sensations of childbirth are that of pain with the way most of us do it: in a hospital, confined to a bed, on our backs, with little privacy, and few tools to cope. That is a recipe for experiencing pain in labor. (Not that people don't experience painful sensations in birth outside of the hospital, but keep reading.)

In movies, TV shows, books, and anecdotal and often unsolicited personal stories people share, we are told one narrative about the sensations of birth—that it is the worst possible pain that a human being can experience, that it's a screaming, yelling, purple-faced endeavor, and why the hell would anyone put themselves through that on purpose when they can opt out of feeling it at all?

First, I'll address the "why." Giving birth without an epidural is not a noble endeavor. It is not morally superior, and it does not mean you're stronger or more resilient than someone who chooses an epidural or is coerced into having one. It does not mean you love your baby more because you chose to birth without an epidural. The reason you might want to feel the sensations of your labor is because in most cases, it is the safer option, not just for your baby, but for you. The sensation of childbirth provides valuable information about the positioning of your baby and what your body needs to open. The lack of epidural anesthesia* means the ability to walk around, change positions unencumbered, and be in an upright position where gravity can work in your favor, which are all important things to facilitate your birth.

....

* The pros of an epidural are that it numbs pain, it allows you to sleep (and sleep promotes the proper brainwaves needed for labor to progress), and for some birthing people they need it to relax (preferably after they're at least 6 centimeters dilated). The cons of an epidural are that it restricts movement. (Movement is still possible, but multiple helping hands are necessary to change positions. It can potentially slow the baby's heart rate, usually as a result of staying in one position). It can cause "failure to progress," which is the way the medical-industrial complex pathologizes a birthing person's labor being anything other than straightforward and linear. Because of "failure to progress," getting an epidural necessitates a medical induction, which is the introduction of artificial birth hormones (Pitocin or cytotec) that increase the intensity and frequency of contractions. These intense contractions can often cause fetal distress, which can then ultimately necessitate surgical birth. One of the less talked about cons of an epidural is that they are fallible (because the people who place them are fallible), which can lead to long-term birth injury. One of the most common side effects of an epidural is lifelong lower back pain.

Also, if you find yourself reading this particular book, your "why" might be something like mine: I, personally, chose to create a whole new human with my partner because I wanted to experience the full spectrum of what the human experience has to offer. I didn't buy into the cultural story that this pain was bigger than me, and I didn't believe it was pointless or torture. Birth is the only normal bodily function that we experience as painful when there's nothing wrong (usually pain is indicative of a problem or an injury in the body). I refuse to believe that whatever the intensity of this sensation, that it is there by mistake. I prepared with hypnobirthing techniques to hopefully make my intensity of labor not feel like pain. And, ultimately, I knew whatever came wouldn't be forever, and I could endure anything as long as it was temporary.

There are lessons and beautiful medicine in validating your choice to numb the sensations of labor. In some cases, and some birth experiences, I would even recommend it in order to let go and release. And there are certainly people who are pregnant and birthing solely because they want the prize of that sweet babe at the end; again, valid and beautiful.

For me, it didn't make sense to plan to numb the pinnacle of this pregnancy experience because I personally came here to *experience* it. I did not decide to climb Mount Everest so I could helicopter to the top just to enjoy the view; I wanted the hike too.

The intensity of these sensations is an invitation to tap into the brainwaves that people pay money to experience through ayahuasca or DMT—your magical body (your pineal gland, to be precise) has the opportunity to conjure that magic all by itself without the help of drugs. That is literal magic! Not everyone will experience this transcendent effect of birth, but we know it's possible, so why not plan for transcendence instead of planning for fear, resistance, and numbing?

Also, it should be noted that even when one plans for epidural anesthesia, it is not necessarily a get-out-of-pain-free card. You'll want to do a good amount of laboring at home before getting to the hospital, so that way labor doesn't slow down from the car ride to getting admitted. And ideally, you'd get to at least 6 centimeters dilated before having an epidural administered because at that point it is less likely to slow down the progress of your labor. Getting the epidural itself can even be painful, so either way, I suggest learning some techniques to cope with pain (see "Comfort Measures for Moving through Intensity," page 219).

When I hear pregnant people or parents talk about their labor, whether they've already done it or not, it's mostly framed as though the ability to persevere through pain and achieve a "natural"* birth is the moral high ground attached, and "failure" to achieve "natural" birth is described with guilt, such as *I caved and asked for the epidural.* Now is a good time to reiterate that there is no right or wrong way to give birth. There are only the choices we make and then what we learn, how we grow and evolve out of our experiences. But this dichotomy sets us up to believe the idea that we're either nobly suffering, or we're pragmatically choosing to opt out of suffering, as if those are the only options.

I would prefer to throw that either/or notion out entirely. There truly is no opting out of "pain" entirely, even if you're choosing a fully medicalized birth. Getting an epidural is painful, being induced with a Foley balloon is painful, healing from major abdominal surgery is painful. I'm not saying that any or all these experiences of pain will necessarily happen to you, but they are possible, nonetheless. Research shows that people who planned for epidurals and got them often reported the experience of their births as more painful than people who planned to birth without pain medication entirely.

My interpretation of this card looks at how much our mindset and preparation have to do with the way we experience sensation. If your idea of labor was that your water would break, you'd rush to the hospital like in the movies, and then not feel anything until your baby arrived hours later, you might be surprised and upset by how much laboring on your own you'd need to do before they'd even allow an epidural, and you might be caught off guard by how painful a needle in the spine can be. It makes sense that if you thought you were planning for a painless experience, then you might find the pain you did have to endure to be unacceptable.

When we see the ways a birthing person's body opens, we consider our own body, solid and closed, and think, *How can that* not *be painful?* But I think this idea is rooted in patriarchal ideology, one that told us that childbirth can only be pain, and that pain was ours to endure because of Eve's disobedience and wantonness. And even in cultures where Christianity is not the prevailing religion, because of colonialism, many cultures uphold this patriarchal ideology of how we perceive the sensations of birth and whether we can or should experience it or numb it.

But biology has set us up with some protection against these sensations being

* *Natural* is in quotation marks because what people mean is vaginal birth without pain medication, when most of the time they still plan for or accept medical augmentations to what would be an organic flow of a normal physiologic birth, such as allowing IVs, allowing continuous fetal monitoring, allowing medical induction, etc.

perceived as pain. In a normal, low-risk physiologic birth, oxytocin and endorphins flow to help move labor along and help us perceive the surges as intense but perhaps not painful. When pushing, the pressure of the baby's head on the pelvic floor is designed to naturally numb the area by decreasing blood flow to help ease the sensation of the "ring of fire" (the term for the sensation of crowning). Instead, the ways we commonly labor and birth do everything *but* tap into that built-in help: leaving home or our comfort zone; having our thinking brain stimulated by too much paperwork, questions, lights, numbers, and other distractions; birthing on our backs and not utilizing gravity during pushing phases; staying in one position in bed rather than getting up, walking around, dancing, or getting in the shower. We birth without the presence of someone who knows ways to help move through the intensity, we put ourselves in environments where adrenaline is constantly spiked by unnecessary fear, cutting off our oxytocin flow, and we go into labor with the expectation that our sensations are going to be painful ones.

If you've ever been to the ocean, you know that when you see a big wave coming at you, the first instinct might be to turn away from it, fight it, or try to bypass it by swimming over it. We usually end up getting knocked down; we might find ourselves flailing, floundering, and panicking, unsure which way is up or down. The best way to approach an oncoming wave, however, is to swim through it. This is true in childbirth in both a macro and micro way: in the macro, truly the only way "out" of childbirth is through, and in a micro way, each wave is an opportunity to lean into each surge, working with them and not against them, allowing them to do the work for you in the way that they're trying to—opening the way for your baby to enter the world. Your surges are your allies, not your enemies, and ultimately, this is how the Tower shows up in birth. Because as destructive and intense as the Tower energy might feel, it's ultimately your ally by bringing about necessary change, and it brings the intensity required to bring a new human into the world too.

The experience of pregnancy, birth, and parenthood is such an abundant opportunity for a Tower-level transition where we have a chance to rewrite our stories if we so choose, deciding what we'd like to take with us to the other side of the transition or not. You get to decide how life-altering you want this experience to be, and my guess is that you're reading this book because you are open to letting pregnancy and birth shift you, change you, and move you beyond your old paradigms and tightly held narratives.

ᕬ THE TOWER THEMES ᕛ

personal upheaval, collective leveling, revolution, uncontrolled burn, uprising,
rebirth, dismantling, intensity, big transformation, reckoning, rock bottom

ᴱXERCISE

COMFORT MEASURES FOR
MOVING THROUGH INTENSITY

Here are some comfort measures that help us move through the intensity of
birth without numbing the sensations of it (or if you're planning for epidural
anesthesia, these can be used until you can access your epidural):

- Minimal talking and minimal thinking: The effort it takes to
  think and speak compromises the quiet, languid, soft, limpid
  relaxation of the muscles and jaw that will help in surrendering to the intensity and lower the perception of pain. A thinking brain experiences pain. When in active labor and while
  pushing, the birth team should keep questions to a minimum
  (preferably only yes or no questions).
- Bodily accommodation: If you plan to alleviate pain without
  the use of drugs, mobility is essential. You need the option to
  move freely to find what feels good and an atmosphere that
  supports you in making these choices and to take up space so
  that you feel uninhibited in following your body's lead. Relaxing the muscles and unclenching the jaw releases the tension
  that increases the sensation of pain. Movement, and the ability
  to feel what's going on in your body, is a safety measure too. In
  a birth that is led by the birthing person, the person doing the
  birthing can feel the positioning of the baby and will often in-
  stinctually move in ways that accommodate the baby's body or
  shift in position.
- Vocalizing: The jaw and throat are energetically connected to the
  cervix, so vocalizing helps not only manage pain but also helps

open your cervix. I've had birthing clients tell me that vocalizing alleviates their need for any other coping mechanism; they didn't even need my hip squeezes anymore. You don't need to be quiet for the sake of everyone else's comfort. Direct your vocalizations low and down into your belly, not high, like you're screaming out the top of your head. Sing or roar your baby earthside.

- Counterpressure: A firm double hip squeeze or a fist pressed firmly in the lower back during contractions can greatly alleviate pain during labor, especially for birthing people who are experiencing back labor.* I recommend researching a video or photos of these types of counterpressure techniques and practicing them with your birth partner in advance, so they feel confident when the time comes to use this tool.

- Cold or hot washcloths: I've noticed few things look as relieving to a laboring person than a cool washcloth pressed reassuringly to their forehead (even more soothing and helpful if there are a couple of essential oils dropped on there like lavender or clary sage). A labor partner can use that as an opportunity to massage the laboring person's brow to help them remember to relax their facial muscles, which will help them surrender to their surges and help their cervix expand. A hot washcloth to the lower back can be deeply relieving as well. In both cases, the intense cold or intense heat can provide a distracting sensation that can take the edge off their surges.

- Hydrotherapy: Submerging in a birth pool or a bathtub is said to be "nature's epidural." Don't get me wrong, you'll still be feeling the intensity of the surges, but it can provide no small amount of relief, and is deeply relaxing as well. If a tub or birth pool is unavailable, a hot shower aimed at the birthing person's lower back can be relieving and relaxing as well.

----

* Back labor is when the baby's position is such that even between uterine contractions, the birthing person still experiences pain in their lower back, unlike most labors in which they experience intensity or pain only during a uterine contraction.

- Visualizing: During birth, visualizations, such as opening into the intense sensations of your labor or a downward motion of a blossom opening out, is one way your brain can communicate to your body what to do and lets your body know you're ready to open and release your baby. Often during labor, we are unconsciously holding on and holding our babies in out of the fear of the pain. How this shows up is clenched fists, a tight jaw, squirming movements as if you just want to be able to escape your body, and higher-pitched screams that come from the top of the chest or throat. If we can visualize releasing, opening, softening, allowing our baby's passage, our brain can tell our body how to not hold on so tight.*

- Partner support: The support of someone during labor has been proven to lower a birthing person's perception of pain and their stamina for getting through pain, even if they are just holding the birthing person's hand or maintaining eye contact throughout their most intense moments.

- Other comfort measures include acupressure, essential oils, staying nourished, and smiling/laughing/inviting the possibility of joy into your birth space.

....

* There are all kinds of reasons why we might clench, hold tight, or resist the intense sensations of labor. So many of us have experienced sexual trauma or abuse that understandably makes "leaning into pain" neither conceivable nor wise to attempt at all. If we experienced difficulty becoming pregnant, pregnancy loss, or infant loss, we might be subconsciously wanting to keep our babies in the womb where we know they are safe. Shadow work and trauma healing are so important before or during pregnancy for this reason, so your wounding doesn't inhibit the birth experience you want. Recommended reading: *When Survivors Give Birth* by Penny Simkin.

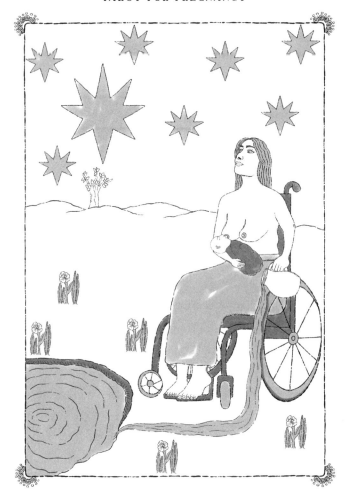

17–THE STAR

"Having helped through thousands of births and literal
YEARS spent nursing and loving people at the bedside, I
have learned this:
the body speaks."

—Kate Novotny, RN*

The Star is all about leaning into the unknown of a dark and unlit path with trust and
faith. It's following your North Star, your light at the end of a dark tunnel. It's the
point in pregnancy where the end is so near you can feel it, but also the point in labor
where the end is so near, you start to question your faith in whether you can do this.

....

* Visit Kate online at www.taprootdoula.com or on Instagram @taprootdoula.

I know a lot of the themes in this book hearken back to the capitalist white-supremacist patriarchy, maybe so much so that I sound like a broken record, but if ever we needed obvious proof of how those systems at play affect us during pregnancy, the Star holds up that mirror.

Modern Western medicine, particularly obstetrics and gynecology, has been built upon patriarchal agendas. Historically, violent, white-supremacist, patriarchal means of study, which were based on false assumptions about the equitability or capability of bodies with uteruses and the systematic criminalization of Black Grand Midwives, are the foundation upon which we birth today in the United States. This is the foundation upon which we perceive what is "safe," "normal," and "right," in regard to how and where we birth and with whom. As a result, it doesn't matter if the people we are hiring to be our care providers within the medical-industrial complex share the same intersection of identities as us, because the system within which they work is thickly entangled with stubborn patriarchal and white-supremacist roots.

If the Star represents feeling your way in the dark, with faith and trust, then it should make sense what this energy has to do with pregnancy, birth, postpartum, and even parenthood. Pregnancy and birth are long paths in utter darkness, especially for first-time birthing folks. Both the person carrying the baby and their care provider are required to trust a birthing person's body with the job of carrying and birthing their own baby.

Within the medical-industrial complex, I would say that often this trust is withheld by the birthing person, the care provider, or both. You might think, *Well, if medical intervention occurred, it must have been necessary, right?* Unfortunately, evidence shows that this is not always the case. Many interventions occur from a lack of knowledge of what is within the realm of normal for physiologic birth, or failure to cater to the requirements of physiologic birth to occur safely in the first place.

Medical providers are medical professionals who know how to do the medical things they were trained to do, so imagine how they show up for a normal physiologic bodily function such as birth. What about when there is nothing required for a person in labor other than patience, reserved observation, and emotional or physical support as requested? What about when all we need from our care providers is for them to step into our unlit path with us and trust in our bodies too? The medical-industrial complex assumes that birthing people can't carry and birth their babies without assistance, management, and inevitable intervention. This is rooted in the patriarchy because it has an inherent distrust of giving people with uteruses responsibility.

It's similar to how patriarchally rooted laws want to decide for people with uteruses whether they are currently in a position to carry a fetus with which they've been impregnated. When they don't trust us to make decisions for ourselves, they assume that they can and should be trusted to make decisions for us.

This can be expounded upon further when you add other marginalized identities to the mix. For example: there are care providers out there still operating under the false and racist assumption that Black birthing people are experiencing worse birth outcomes than white birthing people because of poor nutrition, drug use, or other failures to maintain a healthy environment for their growing babies, rather than the scientifically proven fact that care providers' own racism and patient neglect is the actual root cause of Black birthing people dying at three to twelve times[*] the rate of white women during childbirth and after.

I have seen some of the most confident and empowered friends I know become quick to give their power away once they become pregnant. This shows up like preferring a midwife who represents more of a matriarchal authority figure telling you what to do, instead of a midwife who offers you only balanced information, ultimately requiring you to make your own decisions. This shows up like fighting for better care and questioning everything when it comes to dealing with doctors to help manage your mom's cancer, but once the doctor is an OB, and you're a pregnant person, your attitude becomes *Whatever the doctor says goes*.

It's possible to dig into this void and eviscerate why fully embodied and empowered people shrink in the face of rigid requirements of medicalized pregnancy and birth management.

While all this may seem like flaws in the system, this is actually evidence of the medical-industrial complex working exactly as it was designed and intended. One intervention often necessitates another, and another, and another, all of which works to ensure two things: the presumed necessity of sole reliance on modern medicine to birth a baby (not just when it proves necessary but compulsory for every patient) and the unmitigated, and often unnoticed, additions of procedures to the hospital tab (for instance, after a Cesarean birth, one is charged for skin-to-skin contact with their baby).

....

[*] At the time of writing, the national average of prenatal mortality and morbidity for Black birthing people is three to four times higher than that of white birthing people, meaning Black birthing folks are three to four times more likely to die during or after birth or sustain lasting birth injury. However, in some areas, like New York City, that statistic skyrockets to twelve times higher. These deaths and morbidities have been proven to be preventable. These statistics are true for Black babies, too, at birth and within the first year of life.

I doubt any one single care provider within the medical-industrial complex is tapping the tips of their fingers together like a classic TV villain, gleeful over the enormously successful profit of the medical-industrial complex at the expense of the next generations, but they don't have to. It doesn't have to be any one individual's personal agenda when a system is designed to work a certain way.

I know this is a relatively bleak take on a card that typically carries an energy of sweetness and assurance to it. Positioned as it is after the major upheaval of the Tower, it is meant to be our rest, our coming to a stream after trudging through the desert. And it is still this oasis for us.

We cannot necessarily demand that the entire system change overnight to something that aligns with being solely in the best interest of birthing people and their babies, but we can decide today, right now, that we are going to make our own decisions rooted in our own best interests, not in fear, lack of knowledge, or conventional wisdom. We can decide today, right now, to trust our bodies to birth like we trust our bodies to do any other bodily function, such as breathe, digest, wake up, fall asleep, or defecate. We can do some serious work to root out the ways we've internalized this inherent distrust of our bodies and start cutting cords with that distrust. We can entertain the idea that maybe we aren't as broken as we've been led to believe and see how it feels to try on that idea for a few minutes. Then maybe try doing it as a daily practice. We can educate ourselves on evidence-based birth to learn how what we're currently doing is not in alignment with the actual science.

As far as medical intervention is concerned, less is more. Research the accuracy of some of the tests you're opting for during pregnancy if they are going to play a role in how your care provider manages your pregnancy, research how accurate those tests are, research the evidence-based implications of doing nothing or postponing. Another way we can help dismantle patriarchal influence on trusting our bodies is to listen to normal, unremarkable birth stories where people birthed their babies without emergency, trauma, or intervention and sit with the possibility that maybe it will all be okay. By establishing a regular practice, before and during pregnancy, using education to normalize and hold fierce boundaries around the kind of energy we'll allow into our sphere of influence, we will begin to wear down the century-old idea that unmitigated birth is inherently dangerous.

Have grace for yourself as you go—dismantling entire systems at play within yourself is not light work and we will likely fall back into very profitable forms of doubt or fear. In many ways, doesn't the system consistently profit off our doubt and fear?

Some of us have more reason than just the systems at play to withhold trust from our bodies if we've experienced trauma, or if we have existing conditions like poly cystic ovary syndrome, diabetes, a previous Cesarean, pregnancy loss, or disabilities. These preexisting circumstances can undoubtedly make the act of learning to trust your body's abilities more difficult and you might need to offer yourself even more grace in this. Or you can focus your efforts on trusting your intuition more if your body feels untrustworthy.

The work you put in now will ripple out into the next generation that you're birthing. Keep the vision: Imagine yourself, decades from now, able to be the steady and serene North Star for your child if they choose to gestate and give birth. Imagine the impact your inherent and unwavering trust in their body's abilities and your trust in their own intuitive wisdom will have on their pregnancy and birth experience. This work is hard, but know that the gifts of healing distrust in your body or your intuition has a multiplication effect that isn't just for you.

The Star is not just a helpful ally in trusting your body and your intuition when everything is fine, even when there's pressure to look for ways that it's not fine. The Star is also an ally when something actually *is* wrong, that does truly necessitate medical intervention. I've seen birthing people enact the energy of the Star beautifully and intuitively to demand immediate action, even when their care providers were blasé about the birthing person's sense of urgency. These people were not special or more spiritually connected than you. They didn't know to demand help because their whole path was illuminated, or because they knew exactly what was wrong in that moment, but because they trusted their own inherent abilities of discernment, judgment, and intuition.

It is an absolute revolution to trust yourself with the responsibility of carrying and birthing your baby, something you've poured so much love and hope into. It is revolutionary to do so in a society that is hell-bent on telling you that you are selfish and reckless for making unpopular birth decisions. It is an even bigger revolution to enact this trust when your past experiences give you all the reason in the world to expect the worst for yourself.

While we won't expect to upend the systems influencing us and interfering with us overnight, each and every one of us who does the work to trust our bodies and trust our intuition, and then demands that our birth team follows suit, creates tiny strides toward shifting the paradigm and upgrading the standard of care for the better of everyone.

I acknowledge wholly that not everyone can or is willing to enact what this card calls us in for. It is a tangible reality for marginalized folks that refusing interventions, making demands, or requesting care outside standard procedure can result in retaliation, medical violence in the form of forced intervention, or at the very least being labeled "noncompliant," which can snowball into allegations of medical neglect, making families vulnerable to predatory CPS interference. I am in no way implicating that the impetus of responsibility rests on birthing folks who have been marginalized within the current system.

The energy of Star is basically the essence of what I want you to get out of this book. The energy of the Star shows us how the choices you make around the ways in which you carry and birth your baby can be radical. This card gracefully shows us how those choices, and the standard of care and respect you require from your team, play their part in normalizing a new paradigm of pregnancy, birth, and postpartum care that is centered on the birthing person, rather than centered around care-provider convenience or industry profit.

ᚷ THE STAR THEMES ᚼ

self-trust, trusting your body, trusting your baby, intuition, feeling your way in the dark, North Star, light at the end of the tunnel, rest on a journey, faith

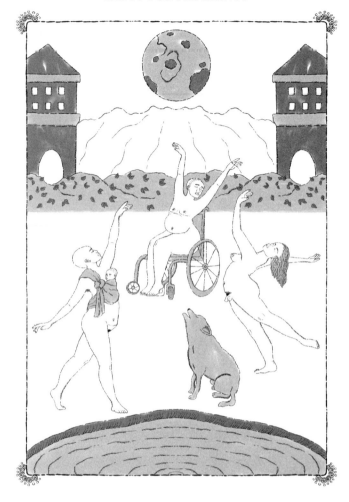

18–THE MOON

"Birth (every kind) is a series of portals + doorways that lead to an outcome. There is no straight path, just illusions of control."

—Davinah Simmons, doula and educator*

The Moon archetype in the tarot represents cyclical nature and leaning into the mysterious unknown. The Moon archetype wants us wild, so this card can frequently denote a suggestion of taking a spiritual journey inward, into our own unilluminated side. The image of the Moon illustrates the truth that all that exists is not

....

* Find Davinah on Instagram @rootedbirthdoula.

always visible, there is information in our shadows, and there is ease to be found in attuning ourselves with the cycles of things.

This lunar wisdom holds so much information we can incorporate into our own pregnancy, birth, and postpartum experiences. When the Moon energy reveals itself in a spread, it's time to pay attention, learn from, and then align our behavior with the moon's medicine. Instead of resisting cycles, we can flow with them, play into them, and cultivate much more comfort, ease, and richness in each phase. Here is how each phase of the moon corresponds to each phase of pregnancy:

❋ THE NEW MOON'S MEDICINE ❦
(IMPLANTATION AND FIRST TRIMESTER)

newness, not yet visible but still there, going inward, quiet reflection, beginning to listen to the inner voice, beginning to get comfortable in the darkness and unknown

Implantation and the first trimester is a new moon phase. It's completely dark and you can't see the evidence of a new beginning, but you still know it's there. It's a time of quiet reflection, inaction, intention setting, and seed planting; a time to exercise getting in touch with the subtle energetic shifts of a new, unknown phase on the horizon. It's a start, a blank slate, a period of work that is likely entirely behind the scenes, work unknown to everyone else but you.

Newness requires us to be humble enough to admit that we don't know everything. Nor are we even wholly known by ourselves any longer. If you are reading this book as a companion to your very first pregnancy, then puberty was likely the last time you ever experienced a new function that your body was capable of initiating and carrying out all on its own without you trying. So, curiosity is a high commodity in this phase, valued over knowing it all, or what you've heard before. Instead explore: *What's this new sensation? What is there to this experience I haven't explored yet? What does my baby have to teach me?*

Newness requires us to get quiet enough to hear the winding new pathways of needs and desires our bodies are subtly trying to communicate to us in a language we're only just learning as we go. It is the work of the new moon to slow down and get quiet enough to hear these subtle communications and hone our ability to interpret this new and foreign language.

⊰ THE WAXING MOON'S MEDICINE ⊱
(SECOND AND THIRD TRIMESTERS)

a good time for manifestation, building, growing, enhancing and honing our ability to
listen to our inner voice, putting wheels in motion, minding your own business,
accumulating information and making plans, establishing new habits

The bulk of a pregnancy is mirrored in the waxing moon phase. The waxing moon and this portion of pregnancy is a time for manifestation, building, gestating, growing, and enhanced intuition. If we can take the lessons of the waxing moon to heart during pregnancy, we can honor that secrets can act as protection—not everyone needs to know what creative endeavor you're working on, or how you're going about it, and it's not the time for sharing anyway.

Waxing is an active time of putting wheels in motion. While you might feel physically energetically low and slow during pregnancy (by the ableist, capitalistic standards of society, at least), it's likely that you're not actually inactive at all and rather learning, planning, and thinking more actively than anything your life has ever asked of you thus far, all within a brief period. Not to mention, your body is perpetually active in growing a fresh new human from scratch, which is work that doesn't *look* like work, but it *is*, and it can leave you short of breath and tired all the time.

The work of the waxing moon is to focus on what you're growing. To practice exercising your intuitive abilities and honing them. To develop and hone your ability to question and perceive the world through a new lens, interrogating everything, to ensure the foundation upon which you build your plans is solid.

It's a lovely time to establish new habits that have a better chance of sticking over the long term. It's a lovely time to lay groundwork in the form of plans and implementing structures.

The waxing moon phase helps with everything on your to-do list, from gathering baby items, to taking childbirth education classes, hiring your doula, and planning for postpartum.

The waxing moon phase has a hopeful, optimistic energy about it, and there's no good reason not to play into that naturally available energy and attempt to cultivate it during pregnancy. Don't be afraid to carefully curate who is in your orbit if they are contradictory to this energy you're trying to nurture during a waxing phase.

♀ THE FULL MOON'S MEDICINE ☽
(FULL GESTATION AND BIRTH)

when our personal power is more potent than ever, things that previously seemed
impossible are possible, abundance, sensuality, sharing, connection and
communication with the divine and/or ancestors, so powerful and intense it can be
frightening but that power and intensity is completely conjured from within

Birth is a time to present what we've been working on to the world, to fully express ourselves, for our purposes. This is the unveiling of your womb's art project. The full moon is a time when what we've manifested comes to fruition and the world finally gets to see what we've been working on.

Our magic is more potent, and our power is more powerful on full moons, and the same is true when we step into being a birthing person. Obstacles that once seemed insurmountable don't need to feel that way anymore. Endeavors that you thought were too big for you no longer need to feel that way, if you are remembering that this you, the birthing you, is a more magical, more powerful version of yourself than you have gotten to meet before now.

If we are fully channeling and embodying the energy of a full moon in birth, we can reach out, ask for, and claim sensations of excitement, abundance, sensuality, and even connection to or communication with the divine and/or our ancestors. But we do have to do the work of claiming those experiences, and we had to have already done that work in the waxing phase to set ourselves up to achieve full moon–level possibilities.

Like anything else that we hope for, it can be frightening or overwhelming when we actually get what we want, causing us to truncate or diminish our own power or question our own intuitive knowing (or perhaps give more weight to external influences who are trying to diminish that power for us). This is a natural inclination, because it is a big, scary endeavor to meet your capabilities face-to-face, and to own that instead of deferring responsibility to someone else. However, it is possible to hold the enormity of birth—in all its overwhelming power and awe-striking beauty— without playing hot potato with its intensity. To sit with and hold what's big, and hard, and gorgeous, and mysterious, and frightening, and awesome without turning away.

As I learned from Tara Burke on *The Witches Muse* podcast, it is possible to shift our view of intensity from "woah" (which halts, pulls the breaks) into a reaction of "wow" (which is expansive and open to what's unfolding). Instead of pulling hard on the reigns of intensity, we can surrender into the awe of that intensity. And the intensity of the full moon, the intensity of birth, asks exactly this of us.

☾ THE WANING MOON'S MEDICINE ☽
(POSTPARTUM)

retreat, withdrawal, slowing down, energetic cleansing, honoring and celebrating the work it took to present your creation with the world, low physical energy, being protective of your space and who is allowed in your orbit, harm reduction, help and support > socializing, rest, recalibration, healing, rejuvenation

A waning moon and postpartum is a time to retreat, withdraw, slow down, honor all the hard work you just did to share your creation and manifestations with the world when the moon was full. Our physical energy is low during a waning moon, as it is during postpartum. This fact works to help you clearly decipher what you do or don't have energy for, to streamline and protect yourself. Now is the time for overdue goodbyes, not with bitterness, but with the calm inevitability of growing apart.

When waning, socializing can feel like more work than it's worth. Honor that. Help and support are necessary to tend to the requirements of postpartum, but not if it requires such a social tax that it's more of a hindrance than a help. The waning moon asks us to recalibrate, go inward, and let go of our need for control and per-fection. Postpartum asks these things of us as well. Waning has a graceful energy that lends itself to forgiveness and letting go, energies that might work beautifully to naturally assist you in coping with and making sense of how your birth story un-folded.

The waning moon phase and postpartum are beautiful times to change narra-tives, noticing how things are done that don't work, and allowing yourself to do it differently, in a way that does work. We typically think of pregnancy as a time for nesting—bringing in supplies, becoming prepared—but it is the waning moon that carries the energy of getting rid of old things, organizing, and undergoing both phys-ical and energetic cleansing.

There is a protective element to the waning moon that also plays logically into what you'll likely be feeling during postpartum, so don't let anyone convince you that your desire for harm reduction is silly or unnecessary. You are the one who is intuitively connected to your own needs and the needs of your baby, and no relative, friend, or care provider gets to supersede that.

The work of the waning moon is not really work at all. It is rest, quietude, retreat, and honoring and allowing the energies that are already present to just be without forcing yourself to be more visible in the world. Our lochia (the normal bloody discharge that occurs after birth up to six weeks) is there to act as a barometer for whether or not we are doing too much. If you are doing too much, you will bleed more, and inversely when you are honoring your body's need to rest, the blood will lessen as well. How convenient and magical to have a built-in doing-too-much indicator!

It is likely that you'll feel more inclined to listen than to speak, and it might feel like it takes more effort than usual to speak your mind and make your needs known. So, make sure you surround yourself with people who don't talk over you and people who make and hold space for you to communicate what you need to with patience.

☽ THE MOON THEMES ☾

mystery, cycles, more than meets the eye, water, the subconscious, wildness, primal instinct

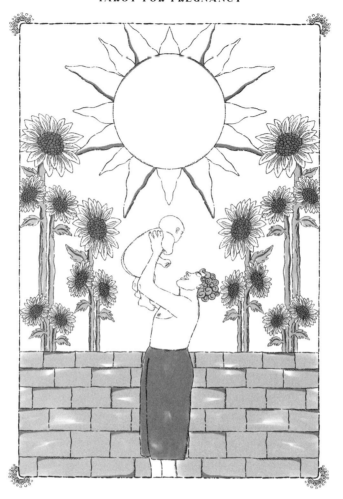

19–THE SUN

To me, the Sun represents the postpartum feeling that everyone expects to have when they think about having a baby. When people say, "Having a baby isn't all sunshine and rainbows," that's because most of us are expecting sunshine and rainbows. And even though, no, it's not all sunshine (because as we well know, there is such a thing as too much sun), some of it truly *is* this joyful, this glowing, this happy, this innocent, this good.

I had a planned home birth that transferred to the hospital when I was diagnosed with HELLP syndrome,* and even though things went as well as they could, a

---

* HELLP syndrome is a rare condition named after its symptoms: hemolysis, elevated liver enzymes, and low platelet count. It is related to preeclampsia but not exactly the same. Because of the severity of my condition and the fact that it can be life threatening, I had to birth in the hospital on a drug called magnesium sulfate to prevent seizures. However, because of my low platelet count, I could have neither an epidural nor a surgical birth, which was thankfully what I wanted anyway.

near-death experience in birth is still traumatizing. When I got on social media and shared that my baby was here along with some photos, the response I got shook me by the shoulders. The excitement, the joy, the celebration, none of that was what I was inhabiting, but my community was there to remind me of the joyful occasion this truly was, despite its darkness (maybe even more so because of its darkness and the fact that I was blessedly alive).

Personally, I tend to focus my work and my advocacy more on the hard and unseen side of pregnancy, birth, and postpartum because mainstream pregnancy books are so wholesome, which often leaves new parents stunned by the Ten of Swords experience that new parenting can be (see page 115). But the Sun's energy reminds you to not lose sight of joy. Revel in the new experiences. Revel in the playful, youthful feeling of learning something new, and playing house with having a *baby* (wild, right?). When things are good, allow them to be good, and *celebrate* the good.

In a reading, the Sun comes up either to remind us to let the sunshine in (literally!) or promises on days that are undeniably dark that the sun will return in the future.

In the body: One factor that has historically produced challenging birth outcomes was that in previous eras the style of dress and sun-deprived lifestyles for the privileged class meant extreme vitamin D deficiency, often resulting in rickets. Today, vitamin D deficiency has been found to be even more prevalent in folks with higher-melanated skin and is linked to preeclampsia and poor fetal skeletal development.

In short, whenever the Sun card is showing up in your spread (and even when it's not!), go outside, or sit by a sunny window, and absorb some sunshine if you're able to. Your body and your baby will thank you for it. Additionally, you can add more vitamin D to your life through your diet: foods like mushrooms, fatty fishes, egg yolks, and the nettles and alfalfa in your nutritious pregnancy infusion (page 55) are high in vitamin D.

❧ THE SUN THEMES ❧

revealing, illumination, joyful radiance, simplicity, clarity, liberation, nourishing but also destructive, less is more

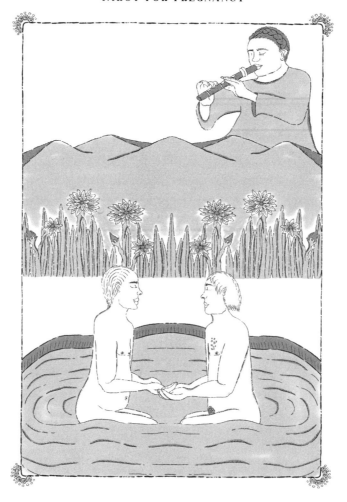

20-JUDGMENT

"To refuse to participate in the shaping of our future is to
give it up. Do not be misled into passivity either by false
security (they don't mean me) or by despair (there's nothing
I can do). Each of us must find our work and do it."
      —Audre Lorde, Black lesbian, mother, warrior, and poet

The energy of Judgment doesn't come knocking on everyone's door in this lifetime
in which they're currently existing, so if it comes to you, know that it is both a gift
and a responsibility. Judgment is when our calling comes a calling. We don't have to
step up and answer the call right away, but it will only get louder, and likely more
uncomfortable, while we put it off.

      Some people do find this kind of calling in parenthood, but that's not the only way this energy manifests. It can also be you finding your purpose as it coincides with the big Tower moment, the rebirth and transformation that is pregnancy and birth. This was my experience, because I didn't get interested in birth until I was a pregnant person myself, which lead to getting my doula certification, led to me being a passionate birth advocate, and eventually, led to writing this book, and uncovering that my soul's mission is to remind birthing people of their inherent power. And I began to chip away at my ancestral debt by trying to undo the harm of my colonial ancestors within the realm of birth.

But of course, not everyone will turn their birth experience into a birth work practice. There are about as many unique callings in the world as there are people, so only you will know what this card means for you when it shows up. Pregnancy, birth, and new parenthood doesn't necessarily instantly wake you up to your soul's purpose either, though I've commonly seen this be the case.

The path to and in parenthood is such an enormous change to your life's status quo that it's impossible for you to not be wholly changed by this experience. It would be impossible for this experience not to push you to be further in alignment with your soul's mission. When this call comes, it might feel scary, or maybe like something you don't have time for, but when we show up and act on this energy, there's no option but to win. The universe, our guides, our ancestors have our backs when we show up for our soul's purpose.

Alternatively, if this card shows up in a spread reverse, or if it shows up and you really don't feel intuitively that it's signaling anything to do with your life's purpose, then it might mean you have somebody to forgive, or somebody to offer grace to. Maybe that person is yourself. Maybe you need to forgive yourself and have grace for yourself in how you aren't able to show up for yourself in your pregnancy. Maybe you need to forgive and have grace for the story of how your birth went down. Forgiveness and grace are enough soul work for a lifetime for some of our lineages.

In this way, Judgment's energy is a beautiful one to invoke in order to help you process or share your birth story. One of the ways I love to do this, if possible, is to host an intimate gathering months after your birth (or whenever you feel well enough) with just your closest, most understanding and tender loved ones, allow them to shower you with nourishing food, and the warmth of their love for you. Then everybody gathers around with tea for story time about how you brought your baby earth side. If you're like me, then your birth story starts at when you found out you were pregnant (or the journey of conscious conception) and everything that went down over the subsequent several months. That story might even rightfully include past pregnancies and losses. So, if that prelude is a part of what you need to process, take up all the space you need. You will be giving everyone present permission to heal in this way too.

It's an important way to be seen and heard, but on our terms, and at our own pace. If your birth was traumatic, this ceremony won't necessarily make the trauma or disappointment go away (and exercise your own caution and discretion with the awareness that retelling has the potential to be retraumatizing), but it's a powerful step if you're ready to take it.

⊰ JUDGMENT THEMES ⊱

awakening to your soul's purpose, being called, self-reflection, forgiveness, truth with a capital T, showing up, ascending, forgiveness, responsibility, grace, processing your birth story

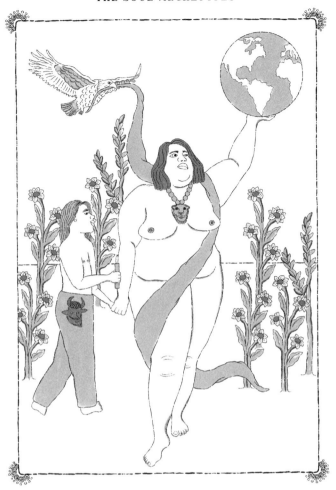

21–THE WORLD

"I am not focused on giving my kids what they need to thrive
in THIS world . . . I'm focused on giving them the space and
support they need to create a NEW world."

—Domari Dickinson, liberation worker at
Positive and Purposeful Parenting

You did it. You did that shit. No matter how it went down, you grew and birthed a human.

Every choice you've made along the way has gotten you where you are. Parenting begins long before your baby emerges, so begin as you mean to go on. Small choices that seem hard in the moment will have enormous payoff in the grander scheme of things. The healing you do now primes your children to be able to do the generational healing that will be theirs to do, a step further than your own.

Sometimes in a reading, this card shows up for me when I've kept pressing my deck for a *clearer* answer or a *more* obvious way of understanding what the cards have said, as a sassy, final, *We're done here, stop asking me questions, bitch.* In this way, this card can teach us boundaries, which even divination methodologies, ancestors, and angels have. Sometimes this card means take the answer you've been given and simmer on it instead of asking for more.

But more often than not, there's really not much more to the World's energy other than pausing to take stock of how far you've come and the lessons learned along the way. This feeling is both entirely full and completely empty. Like the Sun, this can show up as a call to revel in completion, or, depending on the context of your reading, it can show up as a promise of a happy ending (but remember to manage your expectations on what "promises" look like from the tarot).

We (as a generation) each have our own work to do:

- Work to do in the forging out a path to liberation
- Work to do in eradicating whiteness as supreme from our ideologies, practices, and instincts
- Work to do naming, addressing, and healing ancestral wounds

Where I find myself getting tripped up or overwhelmed in parenthood and purpose is in erroneously thinking that I *must* do more than any one person or any one generation can possibly do. I think I must heal/fix/dismantle/liberate the future from the clutches of the white-supremacist patriarchy entirely, and I must do it *now*, so our children may have a pure, free, safe, and pristine future. But I don't have that enormous of a duty. No single one of us does.

Our duty is not to heal it all, to fix it all, or dismantle it all. Our only duty is to set up the next generation a step further in the process. And that is work we *must* do, and yes, many of our ancestors (including our own parents and grandparents) opted out of even trying.

I have the gift of being raised by folks who are older, meaning there's more distance and therefore more stark differences between the generations of my family. I was born in 1990, my mom was born in 1950, my maternal grandmother born in 1928. My father was born in 1948, and his mother in 1910. Most families fit an extra generation or two in the span of a century. All this means is that what was possible to achieve within a generation is more clearly obvious to me.

In talking with and working with my mother on breaking relationship cycles and unloading ancestral baggage, seeing what changes were and are possible from our respective vantage points, it's become easier (for me) to have some grace for previous generations. The kind of healing and communication that comes so easily to me and my partner was unthinkable for my parents' five-decades-long marriage. My sexuality, my style of parenting, my spirit-led work in the world, my relationship—how I live and how I love—is not something my mother could have even *seen* or envisioned for herself or likely even for her daughter, being a middle child of eight on a farm in Delaware in the 1950s. She frequently states her amazement at the dynamics of my relationship.

In her eyes, it's revolutionary that my cis-male partner parents our child as much as (if not more than) I do, cooks dinner, and feels equal responsibility for the state of our home. That would have been an unthinkable quantum leap in progress for housewives of her and her mother's generations.

Speaking for my generation as a millennial, we like to complain about the world the boomers set up for us. But I don't think it was as universally accidental as we often treat it. We have our work. They had theirs. We've played our role in progress. But perhaps the role of the previous generations was to exacerbate the tax on the Earth to illustrate just how untenable it is to live by extractive Western values of civilization while suppressing and subjugating Indigenous technologies that make our human existence sustainable.

Our children will likewise have their own work to do, work that I hope is just as wildly unimaginable to me as a husband cooking dinner every night was to my mom. How my children will live, and what they will do, is not possible for me to envision. It's not my world to imagine, it's theirs. I don't have all the answers to the onslaught of apocalyptic crises because it's not visible from my vantage point in the world in which I was born. I'm learning that what my lineage left me with isn't a burden to be lamented but an assignment. This work was waiting for me, with all the tools, resources, and magic of our specific time here on Earth and beyond.

What work we *can* do is bend our knee, cup our hands, and give our children a leg up. Ask them what they can see up there, and to please report back what's possible. I can follow the lead of the future generations, who will have been born into the appropriate astrological makeup to be fit for the task.

We all have the version of the world we were born into, and we all can chip away at incremental changes until the house of white-supremacist patriarchy and Western imperialism is whittled into dust, easily blown off by the coming generations. We are raising the engineers of the new world—the new world that needs to understand just how old it really is.

What world we leave our children and grandchildren can be considered a burden to future generations only if we opt out of doing our own part or fail to humbly recognize that our own work is not the end all, be all of what's possible.

☽ THE WORLD THEMES ☾

full circle, completion, ending, new beginning, circle of life, fullness, bigger picture, the wheel of fortune but even more matured, our generational work to do, ancestral healing

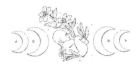

CLOSING CEREMONY

Whenever I leave a birth, after cleaning up the space, making sure there's nothing for the new parents to do, making sure the sitz bath tea is brewed and in a peri bottle by the toilet, and gathering up my own things, I go and find the new parent(s), usually snuggled up in bed with their precious new family member, tilt my head with a bittersweet smile, and know it's time for me to go.

After all the encouraging, tear-wiping, soul-gazing, massaging, witnessing, space-holding, hand-holding, and full-body-weight-holding, it's time for me to let them start to find their footing as a parent. It's kind of like when your kiddo will learn to ride a bike, and you finally let go of the seat, hands clasped at your proud, brimming heart, releasing them into the world, praying that they won't fall (but knowing that even if they do, it's a part of their learning journey).

There's nothing more to do for them in this moment of leaving. It's time for them to figure this out on their own and embark on the journey of learning their new normal. My clients and I just went through something together, something intimate, deeply vulnerable, and life altering for both of us. We went from being friendly but professional (sometimes even strangers, when I'm a birth assistant and not a doula) to being *family*. After a birth I'm always dead tired and ready for my own bed and my partner's healing touch, to go home and hug my own baby and eat a real meal. And yet, leaving is always bittersweet. I'm not always ready to release my grasp on that bike seat.

That's how I feel right now—like I'm peeking my head in your newly rocked world to say my goodbyes—teary-eyed that it's over, but very ready to not be birthing this book anymore, to collapse into deep rest for a long while.

Just like with all my clients, we just went through something together. I know I wasn't physically present with you for your pregnancy journey and birth, but I promise you I poured my soul into these words, so this was my way of being present with you from afar. My way of holding you, encouraging you, witnessing your experience. I hope you felt that supportive energy, even through these pages.

So, it feels fitting to share the words with you that I share with all my clients as I leave their bedside, allowing them to rest and bond with their baby:

I'm so damn proud of you.

Truly, I am.

You did that!

No matter how this experience ended up, whether it met your expectations or not, whether your plans changed or not—you did it.

I don't even need to know your birth story to know that you're a warrior, a rock star, a goddexx, a hero (choose which word feels right for you).

Your baby is perfect.

You are amazing.

I love you. And I mean it.

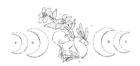

GRATITUDE AND ACKNOWLEDGMENTS

There are a lot more folks who belong on this list, but I'm keeping it brief by acknowledging the folks whose presence or work has impacted me most directly for the purposes of this book.

I want to express acknowledgement, gratitude, and honoring:

To the land stewards, both living and transitioned, of the Anishinabek people whose land I had the privilege of growing up on, living on, and upon which I wrote this book.

To the Goddexxes, my angels, guides, and the ancestors known and unknown in my lineage who support and fight for the same things I stand for.

To the midwives, doulas, healers, and witches who came before me—both of my bloodline and not of my bloodline, known and unknown. I honor and give thanks for the foundation upon which my own work adds another brick, and I give deep reverence to the Black and Indigenous birth keepers who fought (and are fighting) to protect physiologic birth and pass along wisdom, despite incessant colonial attempts at its erasure.

To every birth worker, writer, expert, or mystic who gave me your blessing to utilize your quotes in my book in right relationship. With the exception of the transitioned elders (or those whose fame has made them unreachable) who have been quoted in this book, I look at each of your names accompanying these chapters and I smile, thinking of the exchanges we had when getting your consent, and thinking of the bright, transformative work each of you do in the world. I am grateful your wisdom could round out this book, making it so much fuller than if it were just my own words.

To Kimberly Rodriguez for saying yes on a tight deadline, understanding the vision, contributing the magical spell work that is your illustrations bringing this book to life, and making it richer than it could have ever been on its own.

To Latham Thomas, my teacher in doula work, for leaving no room for doubt in whether I'm going to do what I came here to do, for being a pure conduit for birth wisdom and an example of what it means to live into your purpose.

To my book coach–become-friend-become-publisher, Rebekah Borucki, whose offering came through to me in divine timing, whose wisdom is a reason why this book was able to exist.

To Layla Saad for waking me the fuck up, shaking me, and breaking me open to my work with her groundbreaking Instagram challenge back in 2018.

To Leesa Renée Hall for being a continual teacher in rehumanizing myself.

To Chanel Porchia-Albert for teaching me what it means to center and prioritize intergenerational hope.

To my soul's friend, Kendra, for your kinship that has held me through every part of this book-writing (and life-living) process—from Tower-moment sobs to Four of Wands moments of milestone celebration.

To my Libra sister, Chantal, for starting to plan my book launch party at the very moment I told you I was going to write a book, for everything that implies about you (about us), for every affirming message and reflecting mirror you held (hold) up.

To Cass—for being my kindred companion in birth work, reproductive justice work, parenthood, and sacred rage.

To Tiffany—for being both soul friend and sacred teacher in birth work.

To Rebecca—for your deep, unquestioning, unwavering knowing of the "rightness" of writing this book. You'll never know how many times I drew on your affirming words and kept going.

To my mom—for laying the early groundwork for my love and knowledge of plants, writing, mothering, and taking care of new parents.

To my radiant Kahlo Sol—for being the planted seed that started the uncomfortable, terrifying, awesome, luminous work of breaking me open and illuminating the memory of what my soul is here to do.

To my partner Alex—for supporting me so I can support my clients, for making yourself available to solo-parent every time I must drop everything to head to a birth, for pouring into me after I pour into everyone else, for washing out my insecurities with the brightness of your belief in me and the work I do, for being my partner in parenting, loving, and healing, and for putting up with me for so many lifetimes.